Cosmic Bodies

Cosmic Bodies

The Ayurvedic Astrology Guide to Health & Well-Being

Gary O'Toole

Contents

Acknowledgements

I have many teachers to thank for their inspiration and guidance in the last 20 years. Astrologers Pearl Finn and Komilla Sutton have been particularly influential. Komilla Sutton's classes have been made accessible to me through her online platforms and her work with the British Association of Vedic Astrology (BAVA), which I have been a member of for some years now. I would also like to thank astrologers Visti Larsen and Freedom Cole. They have guided me when clarification has been needed on certain points. I wish to thank Dr. David Frawley, for making the science of Ayurveda accessible to me through his online courses, and Dr. Ravindra Gangwani of MBS clinic in Pune, India, who put me back on the right track to health.

This book was made possible partly through my own life experience and by applying these sciences in my astrology practice, as well as my instruction in hatha yoga classes and workshops. These gave me insights into mind-body types I would not have been able to access otherwise. The teachings I have received for two decades in astrology, yoga and Ayurveda have facilitated my own intuitive approach to exercise. I would like to thank all my yoga teachers and students over the years for their guidance. Carol Murphy and Alexandra Kreis are two such yoga teachers I have had the good fortune to study with. I would like to thank all of the students who test ran the guidelines in this book and Rosemary Foley for her expert editing.

I would like to thank my parents, Ann and Dara O'Toole, for their continued support and encouragement, without which I would not have been in a position to complete this work. I would like to thank Samir Mahmood for his technical and emotional support.

Finally, I have all of the celestial bodies to thank. Firstly, Mercury, which gave me the ability to put fingers to keys in writing this piece of work over the last number of years. Every Mercury retrograde period has added something to this edition, although sometimes it felt as if it would not be finished because of the constant rewriting! For the final piece of work, I have Saturn to thank. It was Saturn's influence that allowed me to let go of this project so that others may benefit from it in its current form.

Obtaining Your Horoscope

If you have not already obtained your Vedic horoscope from a reputable Vedic astrologer or Vedic astrology resource, then you would benefit greatly from doing so while reading this book. You may seek an online resource to provide the information needed here, but if this is what you choose, please make sure you use more than one resource in order to source, and verify, the correct data. If there are any discrepancies in comparing any of the horoscopes in either, e.g., differing rising signs, then please spend more time sourcing your correct chart from an astrologer who will be able to rectify your horoscope for you.

Tropical versus Sidereal Zodiacs

You will find a difference between the tropical zodiac used by most Western astrologers and the sidereal zodiac used in Vedic astrology, which is represented in this book. This is because there is a difference of 24 degrees between where the vernal equinox is currently placed astronomically (6 degrees of Pisces at present) and tropically, as viewed by most Western astrologers on March 21st, when the Sun is seen to pass through the first degree of Aries. This is because our view of this point is actually moving due to a tilt of the Earth on its axis. When the Earth returns to the same position each year, there is a difference in our view of the fixed stars beyond the zodiac (sidereal). This is known as the precession of the equinoxes.

Both the tropical and sidereal zodiacs were viewed at the same position in 285 A.D., but have been moving apart at a rate of about 1 degree every 72 years. The astronomical difference between the two will account for the difference in planetary positions you will experience once having your Vedic astrology horoscope drawn up for your time of birth versus your Western astrology horoscope. For example, if your Sun sign in Western astrology falls under Aries, then it would most likely fall under Pisces in Vedic astrology (unless the Sun reached the very end of Aries as viewed by a Western astrologer). This is because the zodiac is divided into 30-degree Sun signs, and the difference between the tropical and sidereal zodiacs is currently at 24 degrees (2015).

The Outer Planets

The outer planets, Uranus, Neptune and the dwarf planet Pluto, are not included in the analysis in this book. Though they are used by many modern Vedic astrologers in order to delineate certain influences, they do not fit into the Vedic framework of the seven observable bodies in our solar system (the Sun and Moon, as well as the five planets Mercury, Venus, Mars, Jupiter and Saturn) and how these correlate to the seven tissues of the body and constitutional analysis.

Preface

The links between yoga and Ayurveda (the science of longevity) are once more being understood by many around the world. Anyone who has been to a yoga class in recent years may have heard of their constitutional type referred to as *Vata*, *Pitta* or *Kapha*, or translated simply as an 'air', 'fire' or 'water' type. These are the somatotypes developed by psychologist William Herbert Sheldon in the 1940s, which he referred to as the ectomorph, mesomorph and endomorph. Ayurveda has a more comprehensive evaluation of these constitutional types and they have been used to treat and prevent illness for thousands of years. The common-sense approach of Ayurveda is seen in how we now approach any form of exercise. We can apply these same principles to all of our activities in life, be they yoga, gym exercises, leisure activities, or simply our everyday habits and routines. We are beginning to see how one approach to exercise will not necessarily suit everyone. Any activity cannot be a 'one size fits all', but must be tailor-made for each individual. This applies to the type of exercises one does as well as the approach to such exercises. The Ayurvedic perspective of different constitutional types – which is so important when we exercise – is gaining ground throughout the world. It is my hope that this knowledge will someday make it into all of our exercise-based resources.

Just as we know that a healthy diet is good for everyone, we also know that this is too general a statement. Each individual must eat according to what is appropriate for them. Exercises and their appropriate application are no different. Though the same exercise can benefit everyone, it has to be looked at more specifically in order to train the most beneficial way for each individual. One of the many benefits of a daily exercise routine is that this awareness comes naturally over time, though oftentimes only after many imbalances and some injuries are experienced along the way. Until such a state of awareness is achieved, an understanding of the science of Ayurveda may be needed and is always beneficial. Though this book does not cover the ground already well laid out by teachers in the field of Ayurveda, I have included as much Ayurvedic awareness as is necessary in order to relate it to the main subject at hand, i.e., Vedic astrology. When writing a book predominantly about astrology – and its application to physical exercise – there is no way to fully articulate this without taking into account the healing science of Ayurveda.

This book sets out to make more conscious the influence of the planets and its application to an exercise routine. Vedic astrology is a sister science to Ayurveda. It is known as *Jyotish*, meaning the 'science of light', but is more commonly referred to as Vedic astrology. The term *AyurJyotish* has been coined, combining the words Ayurveda and Jyotish. Here we explore not just an individual's constitution, but a depth of study into one's being as seen in the reflection of the stars. I use the term 'Ayurvedic Astrology' to describe the approach I take in this book.

Just as props and equipment help in getting safely into certain exercises in the initial stages, Ayurvedic Astrology can guide us in life until there is an awareness of our unique mind/body type and appropriate exercises and routines. The aim of this book is to introduce the reader to the ancient science of Vedic astrology by using the horoscope to impart an empowered view of your authentic identity and true self – beginning with the body. I have applied this vast and complex science as a tool to impart a view of your nature, life cycles and trends. By learning to go with the natural flow of life, you can make any exercise work for you, as opposed to feeling like you are struggling with an inappropriate activity. I have set out to convey the importance of a static analysis by observing one's constitution in the horoscope. I have given an insight into a more dynamic assessment into possible current imbalances as well as how to address these.

This book is not a manual of exercises. My intent is to share this knowledge with those who already exercise or who simply have an interest in the body and may benefit from this awareness alongside their chosen field. I would like to invite you to investigate the application of these ancient sciences as you reach a more holistic view of your true nature. My wish is that everyone who reads this book will gain some insight into their unique nature, using it as a guide. May the awareness you gain from the following pages filter into your daily routine and may any benefit continue throughout your life.

CHAPTER 1 - SPIRIT MATTERS

Spirit takes a physical body for life experience. With astrological analysis, we can see each individual living out the results of their thoughts, words and actions through their current form at the appropriate time. Spirit's decision to come forth at a particular time is a way for the individuated soul to live out the results of these thoughts, words and actions through the influence of the planets and their nature. This shows the results of actions we have taken in the past which are bearing fruit now. Each individual's constitution is seen at the time of birth in the Vedic horoscope and is the concern of Ayurvedic analysis and treatment. Through a study of your own unique horoscope, we can see how your mind and body are giving expression to spirit in the form of matter. This form is viewed in relation to the five elements as this shows the essence of your life experience. By observing the five elements, we can examine the constitution and the complexities of form in the horoscope. To begin with, however, we must understand the three qualities in all living things. That which is non-manifest is pure consciousness, or pure spirit, and does not come under the influence of these three qualities, or modes of being. However, the influence of these will show whether or not we are connecting to that which is beyond the mind/body while still in physical form.

The Three Qualities

The three qualities are expressed in every living thing that has manifested. They are simply translated from the Sanskrit terms, *Rajas, Sattva* and *Tamas*, as 'activity', 'harmony' and 'inertia'. These three modes of being are pulsating in everything that is manifest and everything, except pure spirit, is expressed by a different ratio of these. This is a constantly changing phenomenon and yet the snapshot of the stars at birth shows the predominant impulse of an individual throughout life. The qualities of activity, harmony and inertia are present in every living cell and at every level of our being, representing the continual unfolding of life, sustenance and decay. When we have an understanding of these qualities, we can see that everything on this physical plane of existence has a beginning, middle and end.

Activity

Activity represents a beginning. It is a quality that is agitated, turbulent and self-motivated. Life, in any form, has to have a desire to be born to come into existence in the first instance. When we start to move our bodies, we increase this quality. In a general sense, we increase this quality by being more goal-oriented. It possesses an outward motion that moves out and to the sides, causing self-seeking actions which can break down into inertia and disintegration. It can also allow the inertia to be broken up and to move into a harmonious state of balance. It is a stage we must move through in order to achieve a state of peace and contentment in our mind/body. For most of us, however, this disturbed quality can dominate our lives. If we never allow the mind/body to settle, we stay in this state of agitation – usually exhausting ourselves into a state of inertia. We may then confuse this inert state with one of being relaxed and at peace. From outward appearances, the state of inertia may look like a balanced state of being. Exercise can take on an addictive quality because of how it makes us feel. This outward drive ultimately leads to a loss of energy where we can slip down into a more inert state. If you have ever over-exerted your body, you will be familiar with this feeling. The *Caraka Samhita* (compendium of sage Caraka), a foundational text on Ayurveda, states that 'one should not practise exercises…in excess even if one is accustomed to these.'

This active impulse is represented by, and expressed through, its principle of creation. This quality has a self-serving component and we are influenced by this impulse according to our unique horoscope. Each planet in our solar system has a dominant quality which we find reflected in our own being. The planets Mercury and Venus are seen as having more of this quality of activity. They represent the elements of earth and water, both of which are more rooted in the world. For example, if we are more influenced by these planets, we may express the qualities of this disturbance by seeking pleasure (Venus) and interaction (Mercury) with others.

Harmony

The harmonious quality represents sustenance. It is uplifting and promotes clarity. It is light in nature and has the quality of stability and virtue. It is the principle of intelligence and has an inward and upward motion. It brings about the awakening and development of a higher intelligence. Being more influenced by this quality means being concerned for the welfare of others alongside our own. When we reach this balanced state, we seek people and things that keep us in balance – just as when we are out of balance, we seek things that keep us imbalanced. Activity and inertia are part and parcel of existence and while we are in this physical body, we are always subject to, and influenced by, these qualities. However, when an individual is predominantly influenced by, and seeks, harmony, then that person is not subjected to the desire or pain that is responsible for disease in the mind/body.

We each catch glimpses of this state (oftentimes through physical activity), but in its purest form, this balanced state is beyond any words we might use to describe it. We may use words like a 'spiritual experience'. Words are mere pointers to the experience we have and cannot fully express this harmonious state of being. Words certainly cannot express pure spirit, which is outside of anything that can be described in the material realm and which this state of balance and harmony in physical form is pointing us towards.

The Sun and the Moon are both harmonious in nature if they are strong and unobstructed in the horoscope. The Sun represents the universal spirit. It is that sense of oneness we experience and catch a glimpse of from time to time and, although words fail us in expressing this experience, we may experience it through exercise or meditation as we put in place the possibility for the experience to occur. We may also experience this state of being through nature or by being absorbed in a task. Any activity where we remain fully present allows this state of oneness to arise naturally. The Moon represents our experience of embodied spirit. Our sense of an individual self is usually experienced through the mind and emotions, as reflected in the Moon. However, there is a deeper level to this that we can access once the turbulence of the mind is settled in a more harmonious state. It is then we can get a glimpse of our true self – our true spirit. We can see this in the Sun being reflected in the Moon, and the Moon then reflected in still water. When we can calm our minds, we can then reflect the perfection of our true nature.

The planet Jupiter also has a harmonious quality, if well placed in the horoscope. It represents the element of space which contains all of the elements – the building blocks of life. Jupiter's impulse is concerned with the natural order. A well-placed Jupiter in the horoscope will express itself through a sense of connection and concern for all of life. An individual who is strongly influenced by a well-placed Jupiter, Sun or Moon will express a more harmonious nature if they are able to express their balanced state without any other selfish desires or obstructions.

Inertia

Inertia represents a necessary ending. This quality of inactivity is reflected in our solid form, which has a definite structure and will one day decay and die. Anything that has a beginning must also come to an end. Though we can experience a state of balance and harmony between the influences of beginnings and endings, we still have to accept being placed on the wheel of time and the inevitability of our trajectory. We live in a body that gives us this sense of being grounded in a physical form, but we must also accept the consequence of a human existence. We may have to agitate the body in order to begin to move the energy and reach upward to spirit. This is why exercise increases a sense of the indwelling spirit as we decrease our more inert state of physical being and our minds become less agitated with movement.

On a physical level, we must feed our body and protect it from harm. If, however, we are only concerned with feeding, resting and pleasing the body, then we never reach beyond states of agitation and inactivity. We must have our feet firmly on the earth, but aspire for greater than what our physical body can provide if we are to cultivate a more balanced life. As we reach this state, we not only have more regard for spirit and its dwelling in the body, but we regard all other beings as spirit and meet that in whatever form it is presented to us. If we are more influenced by an inert quality, then we are subject to imbalances, and the resulting disease and decay.

The planets Saturn and Mars are seen as inert and destructive in nature. The north and south nodes of the Moon, known in Sanskrit as *Rahu* and *Ketu*, are also seen to have an inert and dulling effect. These are known as 'shadowy planets', as they eclipse the Sun and Moon. This obscuring of the light – our true nature – shows a dark quality which ultimately leads us to clarity. However, if we are more influenced by this quality, then we are ignorant of our true nature and our individual connection (Moon) to spirit (Sun). This nature can be seen in these planets, and nodes of the Moon, either as an inherent quality or as a temporary influence, depending on current transits and periods in our lives.

This dark, inactive quality is downward in its motion, causing death and decay, and representing the principle of materiality. However, it also represents concern for our physical bodies in the form of food, sex and sleep. These three activities are ones we need to address if we are to cultivate our energy in a more productive manner, and use the energy in activities which benefit our body, mind and spirit. At times, we may need to protect ourselves by fighting for something or by holding back through fear, as represented by the planets Mars and Saturn. When we are angry or fearful, we are not thinking of anyone else; we are concerned with our own safety. This quality represents the very necessary role of self-protection, but can also lead to thoughts and actions which create a sense of separation from others. This impulse represents the very necessary process of destruction and decay. An ending ultimately brings regeneration and a new beginning, just as sleep ends our day and prepares us for another.

Changing Qualities

Activity can be introduced in order to correct inertia and inactivity can balance the agitation of activity. If an individual is more inert, and feeling the dulling effect, then that individual cannot become more balanced without moving through a stage of agitation with some form of activity. In order to reach a state of balance from dullness, one must move through a stage of agitation. You would not expect to get out of bed in the morning feeling inert and then expect to experience any sense of balance with this heavy feeling. You would have to move your body and wake yourself up initially. The physical body is a more inert form which needs to be moved a certain amount in order to achieve balance. The mind and emotions are more active in nature and need a certain amount of stillness in order to achieve this balance. The experience of harmony is a balanced state of both activity and inertia. In a higher sense, this harmony is an earthly manifestation of a spiritual experience that we feel as a balanced state of being.

Upon rising in the morning, we can feel heavier at this time of day as we come out of a state of inertia. This inertia is a very necessary protective and ultimately rejuvenating period each night. If we allow it to dominate, however, it can lead to laziness and lethargy. If we begin to exercise, this allows the energy to move and break up any stagnation. Once we have the energy moving again, there comes a time when we must gravitate to a sense of balance, and the resulting experience of peace and harmony. This is how exercise can allow for this process to occur each and every day.

Microcosm and Macrocosm

We can see these qualities of activity, harmony and inertia in everything, whether we view them from the level of the microcosm or the level of the macrocosm. These three qualities are happening all of the time, to every cell in our body, and to every living thing in the living world. However, these qualities are seen to change more rapidly in relation to our minds. We can still manage these qualities and become more balanced overall – whatever impulse may be prominent at any given time. Using the body and appropriate exercise can assist us in reaching this state. For example, if you know that you are more influenced by the planet Saturn, then this will help you to make better choices in dealing with a more inert quality, which Saturn represents. Instead of increasing inactive lifestyles and habits during a Saturn time period, one can find balance by cultivating more activity in order to counteract the inertia. This can bring more balance through lifestyle choices. This may mean looking at foods you are eating, the amount of exercise you are getting, or the impressions you are feeding your mind. Ideally, we should all be aware of our daily intake of food, air and impressions, and the quality of them. They can either be more dull, agitated or harmonious. A heavy meat-based diet, with a sedentary lifestyle and watching violence on TV, will increase dullness and inertia. Activity and agitation are increased by eating stimulating foods, increasing interaction and movement, and being more goal-oriented. Balance and harmony are achieved by taking in pure food, pure impressions, and living a more balanced lifestyle for your constitutional type. We will look at lifestyle choices later.

An individual who is strongly influenced by inertia may not have any motivation to achieve balance, and few desires beyond feeding, pleasing and resting the body. This may be a necessary part of finding a new life at the end of such an inactive period. However, if this is the dominating impulse throughout life, then increasing activity and agitating the body may benefit an individual who wishes to cultivate balance at certain times, especially once a more inactive time period is in effect. Though we can always reach beyond a sense of this limited self, there is a very real need to live life and acknowledge the influence of our nature and surroundings.

Awareness is always helpful in this regard and this is where Vedic astrology assists in guiding the individual through timelines and planetary influences. Though you may have no choice as to your nature now that you have already taken a body, you can work within the limitations of your nature at any given time. You can reach your full range of potential within the realms of free will by doing so. Knowing that you are influenced by a more inert impulse for a certain length of time means you have enough awareness to change your experience of that impulse – balancing inertia with more activity if you are becoming too dull. Instead of experiencing the darkness and inertia as something that is oppressive, you can work within the darkness to protect and renew yourself – just as you do in sleep every night. Appropriate activities can be cultivated to get the energy moving once again, or at least until you have more access to balance and harmony. Inertia can be utilised through appropriate resting periods. This will be looked at in more detail when we look at planetary periods and the resulting influence of the three qualities of activity, inertia and balance.

The Five Elements

From the three qualities, we arrive at the five elements – space, air, fire, water and earth – the building blocks of life. The five elements represent the essence of our life experience. They may be viewed on any level of our being, from an Ayurvedic perspective, to an in-depth study of our unique nature in Vedic astrological analysis. The element of space (sometimes referred to as ether) is derived from pure harmony. It contains and organises all of the other elements. During activity, we experience fire, representing mobility and agitation. During inactivity, we experience earth, representing inertia – the grossest of the five elements. From a combination of balance and activity, we experience the element of air, representing movement in space. During inactivity combined with activity, we experience water, combining mobility and inertia.

The three qualities express themselves in everyone and everything, whether it is a thought, a body type, or an experience. Using the body to quiet down the mind is a worthwhile and accessible activity in order to find balance within our unique nature. When we add more awareness to how our bodies function and interact within our environment, we can develop a better flow within this process. We can stop resisting our body by simply viewing it as our physical home without guilt or shame – feeding, pleasing and resting it when we need to. We can be more goal-oriented when we need to move energy, but learn to take breaks when appropriate. We can cultivate a balanced nature and live a life in harmony with our surroundings if we can balance activity and inertia. We may simply observe where our impulse remains predominantly. Though we may be aware of a more harmonious nature with our friends, we may have a more inert quality in our work environment. You may notice if you are more inert, agitated or harmonious in general and in each area of life, as expressed through the houses of astrology. This is helpful in determining which qualities are looking for expression. We can then accept and work with these impulses more skilfully. This breakdown of areas of life will be looked at later. However, the overall quality you experience as an individual is what is referred to here.

The five planets Jupiter, Saturn, Mars, Venus and Mercury represent the five elements of space, air, fire, water and earth. The position, and subsequent movement of these planets in the horoscope, shows our experience of these five elements. Our spirit has taken a body to experience life here on Earth. This experience is seen in relation to these elements, which are under the influence of the three qualities. If, for example, we are experiencing expansion, connection and support, then this is the experience of harmony in space, as represented by a strongly placed Jupiter. If we are experiencing a joyous detachment or a feeling of loss, then this can be the experience of an increase of the air element, as represented by the inert planet Saturn. If we experience more compassion, then this can be seen as the water element expressed by the more harmonious impulse of the Moon. Similarly, if we are experiencing the need for pleasure, then this is an experience of the water element and the active planet Venus. If we experience clarity and are generous with our energy, then this is an experience of the fire element as represented by the harmonious Sun. If we are experiencing selfishness and irritability or anger, then this is an expression of the fire element and the more selfish Mars. If we are more concerned with interacting in the business world and making money or dealing with any other practical concerns, then this is the element of earth, as represented by the active planet Mercury.

These are just a few examples of how the elements can be expressed in our life experience, although we each experience these planets in our own unique way. One thing to note is that when we look at these elements, as reflected in the mind, we must always strive to keep the air element calm. This is the element which creates a sense of separation that can lead to all kinds of difficulties in our lives. Though we do benefit from the limiting influence of air by giving us a sense of being limited by our physical reality, we can experience this restriction in our physical forms if our shape does not please us. We must accept the form of our body and work within its capabilities. However, in a general sense, we can experience an increase of air as a feeling of isolation within our lives, and all the resulting repercussions of this feeling of separation. Often this is felt as a need to be alone and to work on oneself. Balance is achievable and can be found through interaction with others while working hard.

Space

Space is that which contains and binds all of the other elements, allowing them to come into being, organising them, holding everything in place. Jupiter represents the element of space, showing our connection to others and our ability to organise our lives, pulling resources and people into our sphere, feeling connected to everyone and everything. Space derives from the mind, which is itself a subtle form of space. When we experience space, we can slip out of time and sense the vastness of who we really are. Life can be a profound experience and we are uplifted. We are literally given space to breathe. Notice the pause at the end of each breath. This feeling of space creates a sense of peace in life, which is generally the experience of a Jupiter time period. Jupiter shows our connection to others and the world around us. When we are strongly influenced by Jupiter, we develop this connection and eliminate any sense of fear or doubt. If we feel part of something, we are concerned with it and seek to preserve it. This could be seen on a personal or global level, depending on an individual's experience of this element, as seen by Jupiter's position in the horoscope. The position of Jupiter at the time of birth shows where we feel this sense of connection through space. Jupiter represents the beneficial results from actions which were of benefit to others previously. If we achieve anything meaningful in life, it is that we can help others with their difficulties, be they physical, mental or emotional.

Air

Air is that which separates us from each other and is represented by the planet Saturn. Through movement in space, we get air, representing a denser element than space. The separating element of air shows where we feel a sense of isolation. This may express itself as a joyful detachment or a depressing fear depending on the position and strength of Saturn in the horoscope. It expresses itself through the ill effects of wrong thoughts, words and actions taken previously, which came from a standpoint of a separate self, and bears its fruit during a Saturn period and through Saturn's transits. When we feel separate from someone, or something, we doubt it, as we do not feel connected to it. Unlike space and our sense of connection, which gives us a deep sense of knowing, air brings us fear from feeling doubt. Though on a deeper level, we know that we are all one and we are all connected (as air is contained within space), in a very real sense we are living with this sense of separation in our lives. We live in separate bodies, having a sense of an isolated self. This fear manifests in the breath and the ultimate limitation of Saturn is that it dictates how many breaths we get to take. Saturn is known as the Lord of Time. Not feeling the pause between breaths leads to a life without pause. The stress the system is put under can lead to all kinds of disease in the mind/body. The ultimate lesson we receive from Saturn is that we must learn to detach from everything of this world eventually as we grow old and die. Saturn represents the very necessary decay we experience as things fall away in our lives and, as air dries life up, it ultimately leads to our loss of mobility in old age and eventually death.

Without this quality of air and separation, we would not have any boundaries or structure. Even though in theory anything is possible, we must work within certain limitations in order to achieve our goals. If we did not have the limitation of our time on Earth, would we achieve as much in the time we are given? With an experience of air, we can focus, and though at times this might feel restrictive, we must accept the limitation as a blessing for us to achieve anything in life. The kind of joyful detachment Saturn brings benefits everyone. However, it rarely feels like it is beneficial in the initial stages. First, we must experience that we are going to lose everything that we identify with in this physical form. We can only truly say we are at peace once we accept this. Accepting our bodies, just as they are, is the first step to building on whatever limitations we experience physically. With a Saturn experience in our lives, we may experience the pain of needing to let go of something. The lessons Saturn teaches are not easy ones, but they are ultimately the most rewarding. We learn to grow up and take on the responsibility of living a human life, work hard, and, at the same time, detach from an end result. We eventually learn to let go of our self-interest once we have worked as hard as we can, doing the best we can with what we have.

Fire

From repeated movement of air, we develop friction that becomes fire, which represents clarity and is represented by the Sun on a higher level and the planet Mars on a lower level. Fire can either warm us or burn us, so our experience of it is dependent on the quality of our own fire. Our will to achieve a personal feat is represented by the planet Mars and this shows a fire which has more of a toxic nature. This is more of a selfish impulse, which can cause difficulties for ourselves if we push too hard. Our experience of fire can be one of a warm, passionate glow or an intense burning sensation. This is a good question to ask yourself in terms of the quality of your ambitions. Are your ambitions more selfish (Mars) or are they more altruistic (Sun)? 'Mars-type' individuals do well in competition. 'Sun-type' individuals do well in all spheres and in helping others better themselves also. The fire in our belly, which creates our need to achieve a physical feat or mental act of will, is the same fire which shows our ability to digest things. Undigested food stuff creates toxins in the body, just as undigested experiences do the same for our minds. A strong Sun and Mars show a strong digestive ability.

Mars represents our ability to destroy weakness. The strength of Mars will show our capability to get up and make something happen, getting irritable or angry if someone stands in our way of achieving our goals. A weak Mars will make one feel cowardly and afraid of not being able to cope or process the experience. Ultimately, as Mars has more of a selfish nature, it is more concerned with our own protection and selfish desires. However, as fire contains the element of air, it can be seen that fear is the basis of this ambition. If Mars is very strong, or too weak, then there is an imbalance of the fire element, expressed in one way or another. This can be expressed as anger, if in excess, or a need to control events. It may be expressed as timidity if it is lacking. Sometimes when an individual has a weakly placed Mars in the horoscope, they will compensate and may come across as if they have a strong Mars. However, this apparent strength is coming from a place of weakness.

The Sun has a balanced nature so this experience of fire will bring us ultimately to our true nature. Though the Sun is seen as malevolent in Vedic astrology – as seen in its ability to burn whatever comes too close – it is with the purpose of bringing illumination. Mars, on the other hand, keeps us in a sense of ignorance of our true being. Our true power and confidence are represented by the Sun, whereas our sense of personal power is represented by Mars. The Sun's heat is the fire element in its purifying capacity. This can be seen when we Sun bathe and experience its detoxifying effect. However, if we stay too long in the Sun, we will burn. Before we gain an experience of a more confident self, we first need to be selfish enough to begin the search. We must have a strong desire to change things in our lives so that we can facilitate that possibility. That is represented by the strength of Mars and the fire element. Mars represents the necessity to find strength through discipline such as exercise, no matter how we feel in any given moment. The Sun represents a connection to a higher power and sense of self. When we exercise, we balance our fire, experiencing a sense of self-esteem and confidence that the fire element bestows upon us.

Water

Venus and the Moon represent the life-giving element of water and its ability to rejuvenate and heal us. Water is the element which soothes all of life's roughness. Therefore, it can be seen that Venus and the Moon represent the amount of peace and comfort we are afforded. Without the influence of life-giving water, we would dry up, physically and emotionally. The water element is what keeps us in relationships and gives us the need to enjoy life, and our physical bodies when we exercise. The influence of Venus and the Moon grants us the ability to compromise our personal goals, although the impulse of Venus is more selfish in nature than the Moon's. Even though we want to include others in the pursuit of happiness, we wish to have our own needs met in return. However, Venus is not as selfishly motivated as the planet Mars. The position and state of Venus will show this capacity and the ability to enjoy the pleasures that life has to offer.

The Moon represents the water element on a higher level, so it is a more harmonious expression of water. The need for comfort, and to give comfort to others, becomes an altogether more altruistic affair. Here we see a compassionate impulse, without the need to receive anything in return. When Venus is concerned, we want our needs met when doing something for another, e.g., in a romantic relationship, which is ideally based on mutual appreciation. The Moon, on the other hand, represents an altruistic love and a sense of emotional well-being if it is strongly placed in the horoscope. An example of the Moon's influence would be a mother's love for her child and her need to look after the child without seeking anything in return. The Moon shows where we seek comfort in life and where we seek to comfort and care for others. The strength of the Moon will show if this is a challenge or an easy impulse and would depend on the position and strength of the Moon in the horoscope.

Earth

When water coagulates, it becomes earth, manifesting form in life. The densest element, and that which represents our physical bodies and our very practical needs in life, is represented by the planet Mercury. Earth contains all of the elements and represents our concern with practicalities. The strength of Mercury shows how well we can approach life on a practical level. Mercury brings an awareness of a need for security. We work hard at something to become knowledgeable in order to make a living in the world. This, of course, leads to attachment and an interest in developing skills to better ourselves. This could also mean skills in sports or physical feats in exercise. The impulse of Mercury is active and directs our attention outwards into the world. The need to be of the world and fully enmeshed in it is seen with the earth element. Earth is the densest element compared to space as the most subtle. If we get too stuck in the earth, then we miss so much more of the subtleties of life. However, as earth has all of the elements contained within it, we can see that Mercury's influence brings many possibilities. In fact, too much choice can be a result, as the mind grapples with many options. We need to ground what we aspire to in our physical reality for it to be of any practical use to us in this life. Speaking intelligibly and communicating effectively what we experience is how Mercury expresses its strength. Ultimately, Mercury's true strength is represented by the power of discrimination and reasoning. This will vary according to the position and strength of Mercury in the horoscope.

How on earth do the planets influence us?

The influence of the planets is complex. There are five wheels of energy which run along the central channel of the spine, culminating at five different energy centres in the subtle body. They show how the planets spinning in space are reflecting our own being, mapped out in our subtle body. There are also said to be 72,000 circuits of energy moving around our entire subtle body. Of these, there are three that are looked at initially when acknowledging planetary influence. These are the left, right and central channels along the spine. The left channel is the cooling lunar side of the subtle body and the right represents the heating, solar side. The central channel represents the pathway where the universal soul finds a balance with the embodied soul, as represented by a balance between the Sun and the Moon; our true spirit and our sense of an individuated self. These three channels come together at six important points in our subtle field of energy along the spine and then ascend in unison to the crown of the head. They begin at the base of the spine and come together at the point between the eyebrows, commonly referred to as the 'third eye'. Both sides are regulated by the breath, which is seen to alternate between both right and left nostrils every 60 minutes or so, and can be seen to be balanced through both as it moves from one nostril to the other. It can also be seen to be more balanced at junctures of the day and night, representing the ongoing cyclic that nature reflects in our own nature. The left nostril corresponds to the right side of the brain and has an anabolic effect. The right nostril corresponds to the left side of the brain and has a catabolic effect. Activities can be undertaken accordingly. For example, it would be ideal to eat while the right-nostril breath is dominant, so as to properly digest the ingested food. Activities such as the time to retire to bed would ideally begin once the left-nostril breath has become dominant.

Each of the five planets corresponds to the five elements and a point located along the central channel. In Pandit Sanjay Rath's book *Vedic Remedies in Astrology,* he gives a table for each of these centres and their ruling planets. The elements can be seen to become denser as we move down into the lower centres. Space is predominant in the head region, of which the mind is a subtle aspect and is represented by Jupiter. The element of air moves down into the throat and chest and is represented by Saturn at the throat and the Moon at the heart. The fire element brings us into the navel and is represented by Mars. Water takes us into the hip region and the planet Venus. Earth brings us to the base of the spine and the planet Mercury, which represents our more practical concerns, rooting us to the earth. The Sun, representing the Supreme Self, is beyond the experience of the manifest universe and, although the Sun does correspond to the fire element in a higher sense, it also represents the un-manifest spirit which is beyond the influence of the elemental forces. There is a seventh centre located at the crown of the head which takes us beyond the elemental influences and into spiritual realms.

The map of the planets I have given is but one way to view the planetary influence on the subtle body. There are many other approaches. In practical application, the planets can be seen to represent the area of the body which corresponds to the signification of that planet. According to the Vedic astrologer Freedom Cole, 'the natural indications of the planets line up with the nature of the *chakras* (energy centres) more than the elements' (F. Cole, personal communication, October 17th, 2013). So, for example, if Mercury were studied in any given horoscope, though the concerns are practical and relate to the earth element and the base of the spine, the throat is also studied because Mercury represents speech. We will look at the significations of each planet later.

Planets as Karmic Storehouses

All of our thoughts, words and actions are stored in our subtle bodies and show precisely why we come forth into physical form at the time we do. The configuration of the planets, and their subsequent movement, ensures that we are directed to fulfil the results of these actions. They do so by expressing their nature and desires through our subtle bodies, known as the bliss, intelligent, emotional and *pranic* (life force) bodies. These, in turn, influence our physical body, as we are compelled to take actions in relation to our individual tendencies. These bodies are also known as the five sheaths. The densest of these is the physical body, or the food sheath. Subtler than this are the breath sheath, the mental and emotional sheath, the intelligent sheath and the bliss sheath. These become more subtle, and yet more influential because of this, as we look to the bodies beyond the physical body. Beyond these five bodies, our experience becomes more cosmic and is beyond any satisfactory description. Ayurveda is concerned with the individual's experience of self and concerns itself chiefly with three bodies – namely, the physical, emotional and spiritual bodies. These three bodies are studied in the Vedic horoscope in relation to the rising sign (body), the Moon (mind), and the Sun (soul).

Our previous thoughts, words and actions (*karmas*), which are stored in our bliss body and body of intelligence, can be seen to produce results at certain times throughout our lives. In their introductory book on Vedic astrology, *Light on Life: An Introduction to the Astrology of India,* Hart deFouw and Dr. Robert Svoboda state that, 'As these karmas ripen to fruition, they project into the subtle or astral body ...' Once the results of these actions have ripened, we are then directed to think a certain way, which is the planet's influence on our mental and emotional body. These compulsions, in turn, influence our life force so that our physical body is given or denied the energy to live out the results of these through our current actions, or by our inability to take action. This can be seen as played out in relation to the planetary periods, and transits of the planets, in accordance with our individual blueprint represented in our individual horoscope.

CHAPTER 2 - NATURE NURTURES

Our nature nurtures our environment and our environment, in turn, reflects back to us our nature. Having an understanding of the five elements, we arrive at the heart of the science of longevity, Ayurveda, and the concept of the three *doshas* or 'bodily humours' – air, fire and water – as well as how the elements relate to our physiology. The word *dosha* means 'that which changes' or 'that which darkens', a reference to the way an imbalance among the elements can cause disease. These three biological humours show how the elements create our life experience and produce natural tendencies and inclinations. Everyone is born with a unique combination of these three humours and this is known as the constitution. The constitution we are born with does not change throughout life, but we may become out of balance with our true nature. This can lead to imbalances when things do change, such as our minds, emotions and lifestyles. Each planet has a humour through which it brings its influence on imbalances to different parts of our body. The humours work more on a physical level, but they have an impact on the mind also, creating a never-ending loop of feedback between mind and body. When we look specifically at the mind and its nature, we also look at the three qualities which work more on a subtle level, although they are intrinsic to everything experienced, whether physical, mental or emotional.

Ayurveda – The Science of Longevity

Ayurveda is one of the oldest systems of health and healing on the planet. It is mostly a commonsense approach to health. It is a sister science to Yoga and Vedic astrology. Dr. David Frawley writes in *Yoga for your Type*, an easy-to-follow guide to practising yoga for your specific biological humour, that those 'looking into the therapeutic aspect of Yoga are inherently drawn to Ayurveda because of the historical affinity between the two systems'. Ayurveda does not solely view the body and mind in its observations, but takes the soul and its journey through many lifetimes into account – where one has to live out the effects of previous actions. In order to see these results, knowledge of Vedic astrology is required and is why in ancient times, and up to this day, many Ayurvedic doctors were also *Jyotishi* (Vedic astrologers).

The Three Biological Humours

Central to the healing system of Ayurveda are the three biological humours – the air, fire and water humours, which represent the elements as they exist in our physiological makeup. When we have an understanding of the three humours, we can take this awareness into a deeper understanding of the nature of each planet and their effect on our physiology and psychology. Knowing your nature is of great benefit in approaching any physical exercise as well as how you may need to modify your exercise if you need to find more balance within your activities.

Vata – The Air Humour

Air exists in the body as wind that moves within space. Its primary site is found in the colon, but it exists in all of the spaces in the body. Space is the element which contains all of the elements. Air is the driving force behind all of the humours as everything runs on the momentum of the air humour. Therefore, air is responsible for all movement-related functions, such as respiration, circulation and thought. The Sanskrit word *Vata*, simply translated in this book as 'air', can also be translated as 'that which moves things'. On an emotional level, it is responsible for negative emotions, such as fear and anxiety. Its positive expressions are of creativity and originality. The north node of the Moon, known in Sanskrit as *Rahu*, represents innovation and finds an expression through the biological humour of air. However, Saturn is the primary representation of air, producing detachment and fear in 'air types', along with Rahu. The waning and new Moon have more of an 'airy' nature and Venus has a dual nature of both air and water.

Pitta – The Fire Humour

Bile is created from fire, which has its container within the element of water. Pitta represents all transformations in the body. Its primary site is found in the small intestine, but the transformation of fire exists anywhere there is metabolism. All seven tissues of the body (which we will look at later) have a digestive fire. The Sanskrit word *Pitta*, simply translated in this book as 'fire', can also be translated as 'that which digests'. It is responsible for digestion of food as well as of life's experiences. Emotionally, it is connected with courage. Excess fire can lead to hormonal imbalances and negative emotions such as irritation and anger. Its positive attributes are passion and a zest for life. Fire's positive attributes can be seen through the influence of the Sun, while the negative attributes can be attributed to the influence of the planet Mars and *Ketu*, the south node of the Moon. Fire's negative attributes are displayed in a 'fire type's' impulsive nature, which can lead to rash decisions and behaviour. Fire types also have an uplifting and generous spirit through the influence of the Sun.

Kapha – The Water Humour

This phlegmatic humour represents the water element, which has its container within the earth element. The Sanskrit name *Kapha,* simply translated in this book as 'water', also translates as 'that which binds'. It binds the body's structure and lubricates it. The 'water-type' body is the largest body type as the human body is made up of more of the water element. Its primary site is found in the stomach and can be felt after eating as a sense of fullness and contentment. It governs positive emotions, such as love and devotion and, when in excess, creates obesity. It also governs negative emotions, such as greed and attachment. Jupiter and Venus are seen as 'watery' in nature, with Venus having an 'airy' nature also. The waxing and full Moon are seen as more of this humour and are expressed in a water type's compassionate nature. Jupiter shows an increase in body mass if it is influencing the body. Jupiter and Venus together are seen in the affectionate and optimistic temperament expressed in a water type as well as a strong constitution and immunity.

The space and earth elements are found in all of the bodily humours, as space holds the earthly physical body together. Air types have the least of the earth element and are less grounded in the physical body than a fire or water type. Even though we all experience the earth as a solidness of the human form, water types experience this more so, as water finds its container within the earth element.

The Twenty Attributes

There are 20 attributes used in Ayurveda – 10 pairs of opposites. Each of the attributes comes from the three qualities and is expressed in the five elements. Listed below these attributes are the particular attributes of the three bodily humours.

Cold/Hot
Wet/Dry
Heavy/Light
Gross/Subtle
Dense/Flowing
Static/Mobile
Dull/Sharp
Soft/Hard
Smooth/Rough
Cloudy/Clear

The air humour is dry, light, cold, rough, subtle, mobile, sharp, hard and clear.

The fire humour is a little oily, sharp, hot, light, subtle, mobile, soft, smooth and clear.

The water humour is wet, cold, heavy, dull, gross, dense, soft, smooth and cloudy.

The Seven Body Types

1. Air-dominant
2. Fire-dominant
3. Water-dominant
4. Air and Fire Combination
5. Air and Water Combination
6. Fire and Water Combination
7. All Three Humours Mixed

Ascertaining Your Constitution

What follows is a simple table in order to ascertain your predominant humour(s). When filling out the table, you can fill it out with your whole life in mind and take a broader view. This will give you a general indication of your constitution from birth. Sometimes it helps if someone close to you ticks some of the more subtle aspects as you may not be objective enough to see a clear option. If you are filling it out yourself, then do not spend too much time thinking of an option. I have listed each as simple statements for each humour so that the mind does not have to work too hard at answering questions. Simply scan each option and pick the first one you deem to be appropriate. Tick the one that applies to you and that feels right for you. If there are two possibilities in how you feel about something, then place a tick on both if they seem equal. If one seems stronger than another possibility, then place a tick on the stronger indication and a cross on the secondary. Once you have added up all your ticks, you can then add up all your crosses. This will give you a truer indication of type as you may not be a single dominant type. The ticks will give you an indication of your dominant humour, while the crosses will indicate a strong secondary influence or 'dual-type' constitution.

If you would like to get more of a picture of how you feel now, and any imbalances at present, then you may fill out the table while keeping your current state in mind. Obviously, there are some things that do not change very much in the course of your life, e.g., the size of your features. If you wish to fill it out in both ways, then you should get a clear picture of your nature and judge this against your current situation, including any imbalances you may be experiencing at present.

NATURE NURTURES

Please tick the boxes that are appropriate to you.

	Air Type		**Fire Type**		**Water Type**	
Height	Exceptionally short or tall	☐	Medium build	☐	Tall and sturdy or short and stocky	☐
Weight	Light, difficulty in gaining	☐	Moderate, easily gained and lost	☐	Heavy, find it hard to lose	☐
Frame	Light, delicate. Narrow hips and shoulders	☐	Medium	☐	Large. Broad shoulders and big hips	☐
Joints	Prominent, dry	☐	Normal, well proportioned	☐	Big, well-formed and lubricated	☐
Muscles	Slight, prominent tendons	☐	Medium and firm	☐	Plentiful and solid	☐
Skin	Thin, dry, tans easily, prominent veins	☐	Fair, warm, freckles, many moles and burns easily, acne, flushed	☐	Thick, oily pale or white and cold. Smooth	☐
Hair	Thin, dark, coarse and curly	☐	Fine, soft, fair or reddish with early greying or balding	☐	Plentiful, thick, wavy, lustrous	☐
Shape of face	Long and angular	☐	Heart-shaped, sharp features	☐	Large, rounded and full	☐
Neck	Thin, very long or very short	☐	Average	☐	Solid	☐
Nose	Narrow, crooked and small	☐	Pointed, average in size	☐	Large and rounded	☐
Eyes	Small, narrow or sunken dark brown or grey	☐	Average size, green/blue, piercing	☐	Large, prominent, blue or light brown	☐
Teeth	Irregular, protruding, receding gums	☐	Medium, yellowish	☐	Big, white and strong	☐
Lips	Small, thin, narrow and tight	☐	Average	☐	Big and full	☐
Sweat	Minimal, poor circulation	☐	Profuse, strong smell	☐	Moderate, pleasant smell	☐
Temperature Pref.	Craves warmth	☐	Loves coolness	☐	Dislikes cold	☐

COSMIC BODIES

	Air Type		Fire Type		Water Type	
Sleep	Light, tendency towards insomnia	☐	Sound but short	☐	Deep, plenty, slow to wake	☐
Dreams	Moving, restless, flying and falling	☐	Colourful, passionate, conflict	☐	Emotional, watery, romantic	☐
Elimination	Irregular, often constipated with hard and dry stools	☐	Regular, loose stools	☐	Slow, plentiful and heavy	☐
Activities	Always doing many things, always in a hurry. Fidgety, artistic pursuits, travelling	☐	Motivated, goal-seeking, competitive	☐	Slow, steady, relaxed	☐
Endurance	Expends energy quickly, starts and stops quickly	☐	Intolerant of heat	☐	Good stamina	☐
Speech	Talks fast, erratic	☐	Sharp, clear and argumentative	☐	Slow, definite	☐
Thinking	Many ideas, but more thoughts than deeds	☐	Precise, logical. Good planner	☐	Calm and slow	☐
Memory	Learns and forgets quickly	☐	Sharp, clear and quick	☐	Slow to learn, but never forgets	☐
Deep Beliefs	Changes frequently according to mood	☐	Strong convictions	☐	Deep steady beliefs, not easily changed	☐
Emotional tendencies	Fearful, anxious and nervous	☐	Angry, judgemental, critical	☐	Greedy, possessive, sentimental	☐
Work	Creative	☐	Intellectual	☐	Caring	☐
Lifestyle	Erratic	☐	Busy, plans and achieves much	☐	Steady but may be stuck in a rut	☐
Appetite	Variable, erratic	☐	Strong, sharp, always hungry	☐	Constant, low	☐
Disease tendency	Nervous disorders, arthritis, pain	☐	Inflammatory diseases, infections	☐	Respiratory diseases, oedema	☐
Totals		☐		☐		☐

Air Type Key Attributes

Thin/ Curly, dry hair/ Cool, dry skin / Hyperactive/ Moody/ Vivacious/ Eats and sleeps at all hours/ Imaginative/ Nervous disorders/ Constipation/ Enthusiastic, infectious energy/ Sensitive/ Learns and forgets quickly/ Cramps/ Anxiety/ Rebellious

Fire Type Key Attributes

Medium/ Fair, thin hair/ Warm, ruddy, perspiring skin/ Acne, moles and freckles/ Orderly, efficient/ Intense/ Does not miss a meal/ Lives by the clock/ Perfectionist/ Competitive/ Critical/ Irritable/ Short tempered/ Ambitious

Water Type Key Attributes

Heavyset/ Thick, wavy hair/ Cool, thick, pale and oily skin/ Slow, graceful/ Relaxed/ Slow to anger/ Eats slowly/ Sleeps long, heavily/ Affectionate/ Obesity/ Allergies/ Forgiving and tolerant/ Compassionate/ Attached/ Greedy/ Lazy

Dual and Mixed Types

If you are a dual type, then look at the attributes of both the humours, e.g., an air and fire dual type may have a mix of a predominant air type's dark skin and a predominant fire type's fair skin, which may result in somewhat tanned skin that freckles and burns easier than a pure air type. Use this information to enquire into your own nature before looking at those around you. You will, in time, be able to ascertain an individual's general type by their appearance and behaviour alone.
No matter what type you identify with, it would be beneficial to read all of the types for a greater understanding of the three humours as we all have each of these in our constitution in differing ratios. A suggested approach to physical exercise for each type is given subsequently.

Air Types

Air-dominant individuals display the characteristics of wind as this is how the element of air exists in space. They are light, dry and unpredictable in their movement – just like

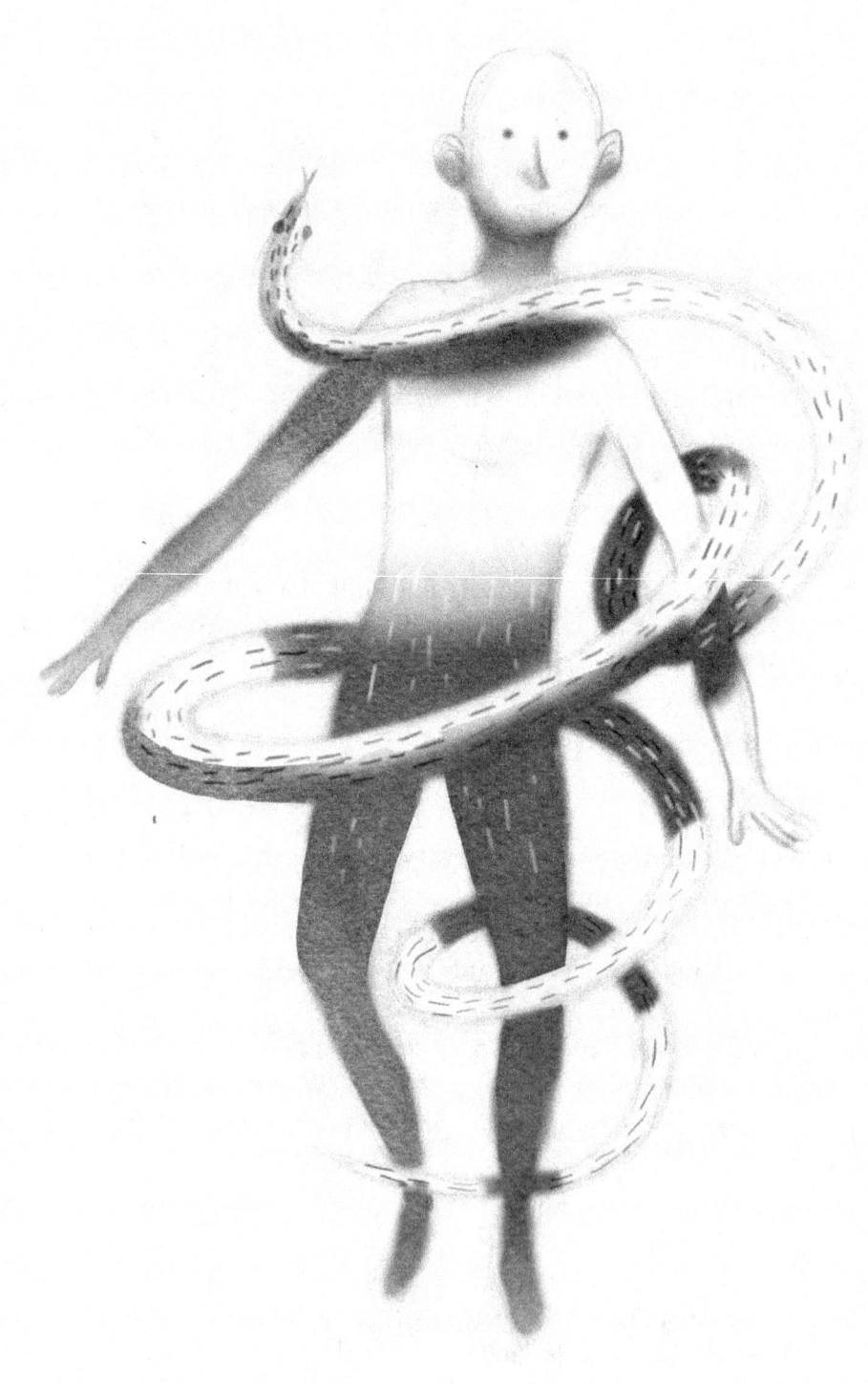

the wind. In order for them to find balance, they must find routines to regulate their system. A daily physical routine that is done at the same time every day is the best thing for them. However, this is not what they would like to do, especially if there is an excess and imbalance of air. An exercise routine offers them a solid foundation to experience the thrills and spills they desire. Their energy is infectious and can come in a burst that dies down as quickly as it started. This must be acknowledged in order to find balance.

Physically, they are usually either very tall or very short. Their pulse is likened to a snake – quick and slithering. There is something irregular about their bodies and their lifestyles, and this irregularity is seen in everything relating to the unpredictable nature of the wind. For example, this might be expressed as an irregular trunk-to-leg proportion. They usually have the longest limbs of any type if the opposite is not expressed, which leads to a very short individual. They are usually very thin and find it difficult to gain weight. This is due to the predominance of the air element being light in nature and its drying effect on the tissues. They are dark in colour and have the smallest frames and features. They brown easily in the sun and have coarse, dry hair and skin. The wind can lead to drying of the external and internal skin, where dry skin and constipation are a result. Keeping the body moist and well lubricated is important for them as is keeping themselves safe and warm. When air is imbalanced, there is fear and anxiety.

Air types are sensitive to everything around them. They do not have a protective layer to buffer them from the outside world. They may feel what another is feeling and think they know what another is thinking. They are like a live wire, not having the insulation to protect them from sensing too much. They are highly sensitive and over-exposed. The air element is an element that separates so they usually find it easier to detach themselves, going for marathon runs, hiking for hours and generally keeping themselves on the move. The planet Saturn and the 'shadowy planet' *Rahu* both represent the air element and this tendency to detach and a need to roam. They need to work more on holding onto things, whether this is food, relationships, work, ideas, beliefs, or the forms of exercise that suit their constitution. They are good at starting something, but not so keen to follow through and complete a task. Their minds are usually in the future and not in the past as much, unless there is a blockage to air's nature, i.e., movement. They prefer to keep moving and this makes them very creative. This future-oriented nature is also the reason they suffer from fear and anxiety. In any daily routine, the goal should be to stay present and grounded in their body.

Air types benefit greatly from slow exercises such as yoga or martial arts. This slows them down and grounds them in their bodies. Any steady-paced activity or exercise is best for them, although they may wish to rush everything they do. A steady weight-training programme will give them the strength they need as long as they balance this with proper stretching. Their irregular frames make them adept at the more advanced yogic postures that other types find more difficult. When in balance, air types are the most flexible. However, they must learn to reign in the tendency to over-extend, whether this is in physical activity or in their lives in general. Over-extending can lead to the opposite effect of creating stiffness through injury and exhaustion. Because our lives are always reflected in the exercise we do, the tendency for an air type is to want to spend all their energy in a frantic dash to the finishing post. They do not have the endurance of the other types and should be aware of this, allowing for breaks and a conservation of energy throughout any exercise routine.

They have the ability to be very flexible, but need to work more on finding strength. It is important for them to remain flexible, of course, because the tendency for them will be to accumulate stress in the body and become stiff over time. This is because of the influence of Saturn and the north node, Rahu, both of which create the most stress in our lives. An air-dominant individual experiencing fear would find it more difficult to find balance with the increase of air than a fire or water type would. They do well by incorporating a slow, daily physical exercise into their busy lives, including regular massages in order to prevent stress from accumulating. Practices such as yoga or martial arts create more space in our bodies and allow the sometimes frantic experience of air to be calmed, tuning into the deeper element of space. Air takes us out of a sense of space and brings awareness of movement and of the passing of time which is, in and of itself, stressful.

It is not usually possible for an air type to just sit still without doing some physical activity first. After the nervous system has been relaxed, and a state of ease can be felt in the mind/body, they can then learn to sit for longer periods. This would otherwise be a challenge for a pure air type who can be seen to be twitching. Air types have busy minds so in order for them to focus, it is best for them to develop endurance and concentration in physical and mental disciplines. Otherwise, they can just get too caught up in planning their future or worrying about the effects of the past and its influence on their future. A meditation practice, or any type of meditative discipline that focuses on an object, is beneficial in helping them develop this concentration. Air type's nervous energy *is* energy and cannot be destroyed, only transformed. A regular physical practice of some kind is the best way to facilitate this. Using this nervous energy in a more energetic exercise programme is useful with the aim of slowing down and conserving as much energy as possible. Though it is not in their nature to conserve and they may feel a little out of sorts by holding onto excess energy, there is always ample opportunity in their life to spend energy. If breaks are needed for this conservation, do not allow a teacher or class situation to stretch you too far.

Air is the driving force behind all of the humours so it must remain working properly for all of the bodily humours to run properly. If the system is put under stress, then air goes out of balance and can subsequently send any of the other humours out of balance. Sticking to a regular routine is the best way to remain healthy. The result is a relaxed mind and body.

Fire Types

Fire types are the bilious types as bile is how fire, and a secondary water element, exists in the body. This shows a hot constitution and there is the ability to perceive and achieve a lot in life. When there is too much heat in the body, there is a need to control. This can be seen in their need to control others, and their own lives, through constant scheduling and planning. They are the most efficient types and need to find logic in everything, but this in itself is like a form of violence – pushing opinions into a more rigid pattern for quick assimilation. This is seen in the hot planet Mars, which is very logical and efficient. 'Mars-type' individuals see things as either black or white. The benefit of this is the ability to pick something that works and sticking to it. However, when there is an excess of heat, it can also manifest as irritability and anger when under stress.

They need to work at cooling and releasing any build-up of heat. They would benefit from a more 'allowing' approach to whatever exercise they plan for their lives. They have the most athletically fit body type so competitive sports such as running or weight-lifting may be more attractive to them. This is not to say that they should deny their nature, as no one should. However, like attracts like, and if there is a predominance of fire in someone's constitution, there is more of a likelihood of them attracting more heat into their lives. In order to balance this tendency, it would be more beneficial to follow a lifestyle that can counteract this. This is true of whatever type you are. A fire type would benefit from a softer approach and less of a competitive environment, as is found in gymnasiums or in competition. A more relaxed class, or cooler outdoor activities, would assist in balancing a fire type. Water sports or winter sports may suit, depending on how dominant fire is in the constitution.

They have the ability to digest large amounts. This is true, not just in terms of food, but also in terms of life experiences. In order to be healthy, we need to be able to digest all that life has to offer us. Indigestion is at the root of many diseases. Fire types achieve

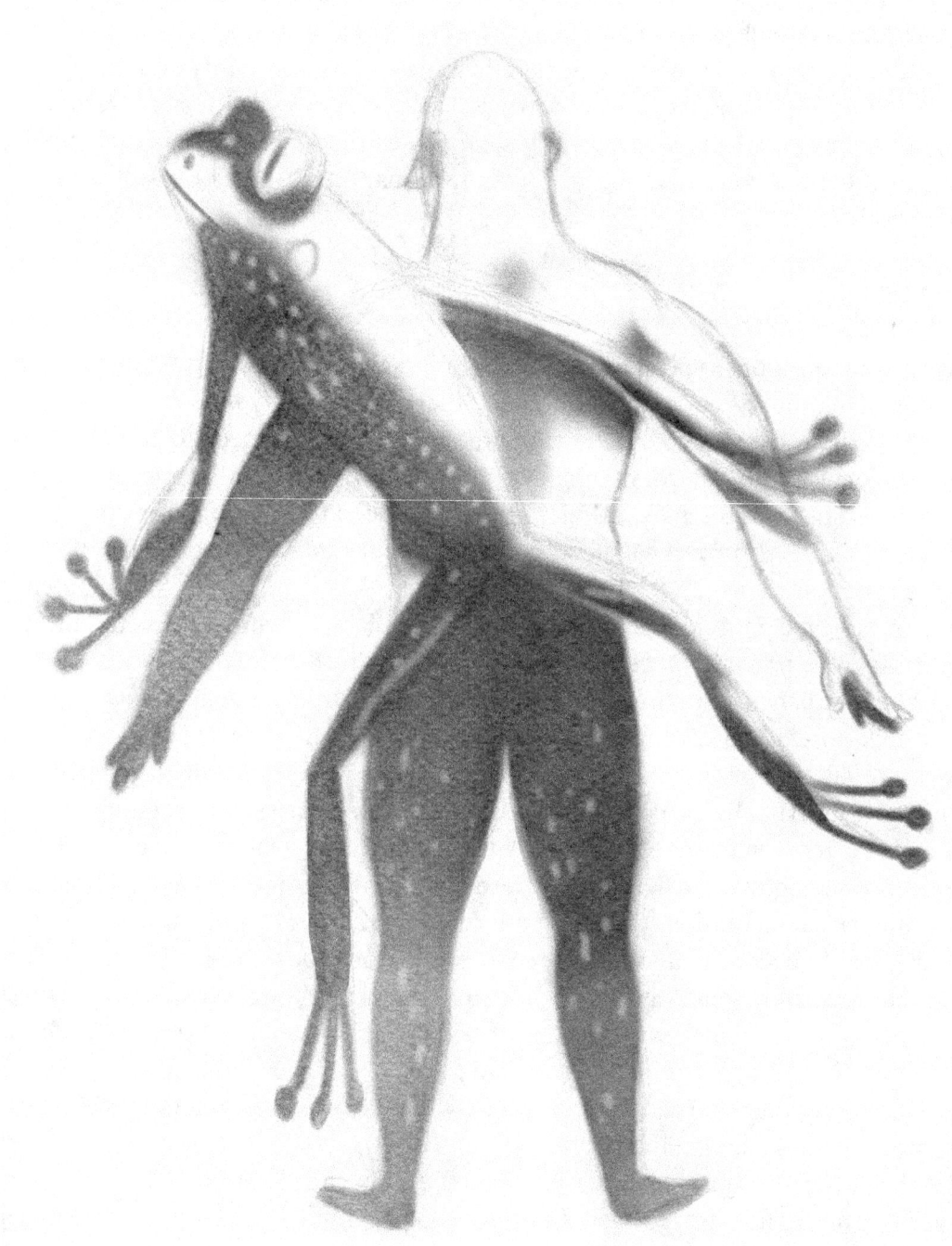

much in life because they have a great digestive capacity and hunger for experience as well as the ability to process their experiences. If there is a very strong fire constitution, then this should not be a problem. However, if fire is afflicted in some way, there can be an imbalance in these abilities. This is reflected in an afflicted Mars.

Physically, they are medium in stature and have medium-size features. In terms of proportion, they are seen to fall in between both air and water types. Their pulse is likened to a frog – bounding and forceful. They have good muscle mass as seen in strong 'Mars-types' who are naturally geared towards competition. Their skin colour is light and they have freckles and moles. They burn easily in the sun and, when out of balance, they suffer from burning sensations in general. This may lead to fevers, infections and inflammations. Anger is present when there are indications of an excess. They have light-coloured eyes that are sensitive to the sun and light-coloured, thin hair that turns grey or falls out early in life.

They are good at applying themselves to an exercise programme, but the tendency here is to have an all-or-nothing approach. They can view things as black or white and would benefit from developing a softer approach to their exercise regime and their lives in general, although they will need to find an outlet for their ambitions and their competitive streak. Adhering to a fire-balancing approach (which follows) will help them experience greater ease and this will have a knock-on effect in their lives.

Fire types have a well-developed musculature which can allow them to work on physical activities that require more strength than an air type is able to muster. Though they have better endurance than air types, they do not have as much as water types, so allowing for this and not pushing too hard for too long is best for them. Tension can build up in the body if there is too much competitiveness. Holding back a bit is always advisable for this type, considering that fire types are more prone to injury than any other type. This is the influence of Mars and *Ketu*, both fiery and impulsive in nature, causing accidents. Cultivating a more allowing approach to exercise will cool them down, yet still spend some of the build-up of heat that can accumulate. Mars types need some physical expression and they benefit greatly by a daily exercise programme, but the ultimate goal would be to let go of the tension that can arise from competition. Meditation will cool down a fire type like nothing else. They are good at applying themselves to a meditation practice as they have the concentration and determination to succeed. To relieve the stress of their determination, it would be beneficial for them to follow a softer approach through practices such as mindfulness, which allows everything to simply be as it is. However, seated meditation practices in and of themselves may not offer them the physical workout they crave. You will often hear fire types refer to the extreme sports and risking-taking ventures as meditative, and may be a better use of their skill set.

Water Types

Water types have a dominance of the water element in their nature and, as the body is mostly made up of water, we see this being expressed in a large body type. Having a denser element in their constitutional makeup shows attachment issues arise, as water gathers in earth. Whereas air types have no problem letting go and moving on, water types like to hold on. This may be to food, people, situations, or exercises that are outworn and inappropriate. They have a slower constitution and more fat than the other types. Emotionally, they are more sentimental and like to reminisce. This inability to let go can lead to a feeling of being stuck, whether in exercise regimes or life in general.

The planet Venus along with the waxing and full Moon represent the water element, showing a need for comfort and a tendency towards emotional attachment. The planet Jupiter represents the vacuum of space which gathers all the elements together, so it is seen as more water-dominant in its constitution. Jupiter prominently placed in the horoscope produces a large body type. The water type is adept at organisation and has great intuitive abilities owing to Jupiter's influence. These individuals feel the protection of Jupiter in their lives. They have a tendency to flow like the swan and can glide through life gracefully with the blessings of the most benevolent planets Jupiter, Venus and the full Moon. Air types tend to be in the future in their minds, creating anxiety. Fire types can be more present. This may fluctuate for fire types if something is not working out as they wish. They may move back or forward to see where things went wrong, or where they may go wrong in the future. This leads to a need to control or, at least, to have some sense of control in their lives. Water types, on the other hand, spend more time in the past, creating attachments to the way things were. Learning to let go and moving on is a life lesson for this type. They can find this sense of moving in a strong physical exercise regime where they can develop the much-needed detachment.

Physically, they have the most solid body of the three types and have the best endurance as a result. This means they can apply themselves to any physical activity and stay with it longer once they have started. The work for this type is to get started in the first place. Because they have more of a slow and solid system, they do not feel light or fiery like the pure air or pure fire types, and do not generally get going as easily initially. This can be more of an issue first thing in the morning when a more inert quality dominates and a water type finds it hard to get out of bed. With the awareness of their

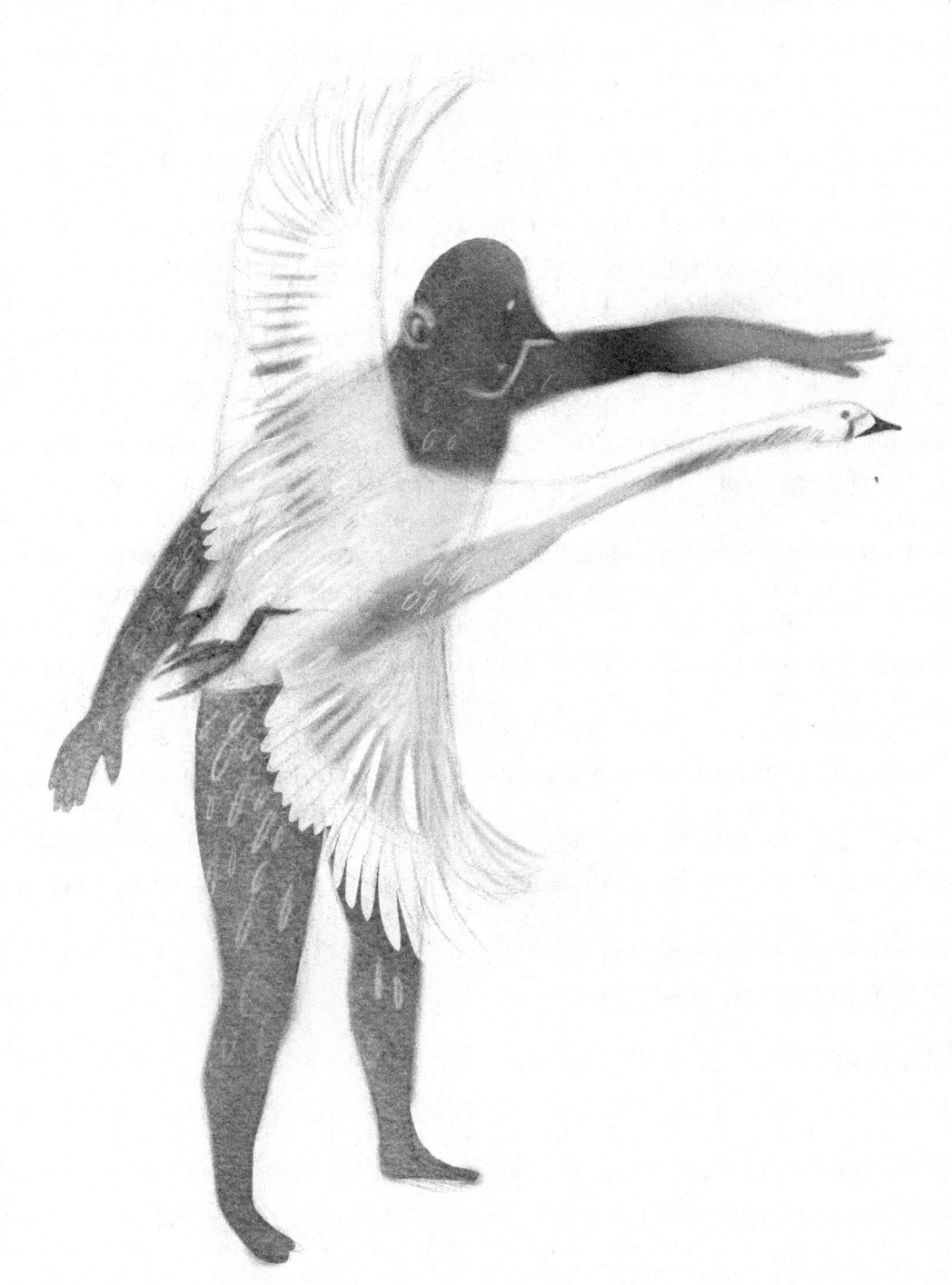

immense reserves and staying power, they can, once started, stay for the long haul. The trick for them is to constantly prompt themselves into movement. It is more beneficial for them to encourage themselves to get over the first hurdle, knowing that once started, they can last the distance. Practically, this may mean staying with a class or instructor who can keep encouraging them towards action. However, ultimately, they must find this in themselves in order to find balance. That is not to say that they should become just like an air or fire type. Whatever type you are is your nature. However, finding an opposing quality to your inherent nature will help to keep you in balance. Like increases like, so the tendency is to be attracted to those things that imbalance you further if you are already out of balance. This is no different when it comes to exercise.

Physically, they are usually short and stocky or tall and sturdy. They have the biggest frames and features of any of the three types and have thick, oily skin and hair, and usually big blue or brown eyes. Their pulse is likened to a swan – slow and graceful. Their limbs are usually the shortest and thickest so they are not as adept at yogic postures, or the more adaptive physical exercises, as a pure air type would. This does not mean they cannot practice yoga and the same yogic postures to achieve physical balance. In fact, a more dynamic yoga practice may be just what they need to remain healthy as this offers the full range of body motion and adaptability they need to stay in balance. They may, however, have to modify the yogic postures to suit their frames. Sometimes, props are used to this end. Yoga may be a more suitable exercise for them than cycling, for example, as this is a seated exercise and does not challenge water types to remain fully adaptable throughout. Not that any exercise should be discredited. However, when cycling (even long distances), the full range of body motion is not activated and water types may never find the balance they need. They have the strength and endurance for exercise that other types find challenging. Their tendency to feel stuck is what must be balanced with their innate strength. In their exercises, it is more beneficial for them to develop a feeling of lightness and to keep the body moving as well as staying longer and working harder at more strenuous exercises.

Dual Types

Having a mix of two humours is common and can be referred to as dual types. When only one humour dominates in an individual, then it is clear to recognise this from the descriptions given, but when two are present, they both mix things up and can be expressed in various ways. This is more clearly seen in a horoscope and the planets, which influence the constitution.

Air/Fire Types

Both air and fire have lightness in common, with less water in their constitution. Of course, we all have each of these humours present as we need all of them to exist in physical form. However, having a dominant type or dual nature shows more of that humour present. It is easy to see an air/fire type by their light body and a feeling of lightness overall. Air and fire coming together can be explosive, so this type must work at keeping the air element under control in order to keep the fire element balanced also. Air is the governing humour as everything moves on the movement of air, contained in space.

Air can manifest as anxiety when there is an excess and fire can manifest as anger when the fire is fanned by air. This shows in their nature as either wanting to control things or avoiding them completely out of fear. Fear and anger alternate in these individuals, depending on the circumstances. We see an all-or-nothing approach and a need for stability as they have less of the comfort of water in their constitution. They may find this comfort in other people or in substances. For this reason, this type can sink into a dependency on drugs and alcohol in order to find this comfort to block out the harshness of life. What they seek is the milk of human kindness. As the malevolent planets – Saturn, Mars and the nodes of the Moon – determine their nature, they lack the more affectionate qualities of the benevolent planets – Jupiter, Venus and the Moon. This will be reflected back at them in life and why they are attracted to the softer influences of the water humour, as seen in Jupiter, Venus and the Moon, in order to find balance. Unfortunately, this can take the form of pleasure seeking through substance abuse. Ultimately, they must cultivate compassion for themselves and others as well as a sense of trust in life. It is always a possibility that there is a need to control things so that they will not have to feel the fear or anger. They must develop a sense of allowing life to just happen, keeping their hearts open despite the mistrust they naturally have of life and of others.

In their routines, they need to develop what water types have naturally, i.e., the ability to stay with activities longer in order to feel more balanced. This does not mean overdoing it or exhausting themselves through activities. It may simply mean being consistent with a routine over longer periods of time. An air type's need for excitement and a fire type's need for achievement make them a force to be reckoned with. However, such highs cannot be sustained indefinitely. This can show up as extremes, which, if at all possible, should be avoided. This can be cultivated in a daily, considered approach to exercise. This type could also practise according to how he or she feels at any given time with these alternating energies. When it is cold and windy outside and there is a feeling of anxiety or of just doing too much, then approach any activity with balancing air in mind. When it is hot out and there is a feeling of irritability present or an urgent need to control, then balancing fire may be kept in mind. Ultimately, every type must be aware of each of these energies and work with all of them throughout life.

Fire/Water Types

This type has the steadiness of water and the drive of fire to keep them going. When these two energies are present, this is an individual who can achieve much in life and with apparent ease. They have the drive of fire and the protection of water at their disposal. They have the most robust constitution and can be quite a force to be dealt with. Unlike air/fire types who have all the energy and possibilities, but who may need to ground it in something lasting, this type can apply themselves consistently. They sometimes need the encouragement to get going, especially if water is more dominant and out of balance. If fire is more dominant, this is usually not a problem and they can apply themselves to whatever they put their minds to. As air is lacking, they must learn to cultivate adaptability in their lives and this is also true in the exercise they choose. Learning to change with the seasons, with age, and with life circumstances is a lesson for them. Learning to let go and detach from a desired outcome is another important lesson in balance. All of these can be cultivated in an exercise programme, or simply making routines more adaptive.

Dual types would ideally exercise according to how they are feeling and the time of year as well as their stage of life. Fire is dominant in the middle portion of life when we are at our most ambitious. It is highest in summer after its accumulation in the spring so exercise should reflect the need to balance this. Water is dominant in early life and the late winter months and into early spring. In nature, this can be seen as the ice slowly beginning to melt. Allowing for this process to occur within us is best. It is happening anyway, but when we have this awareness, we can help it along as opposed to obstructing the natural flow. Air is dominant in the latter stages of life, when we begin to dry out and recede from the world, as well as during the autumn and early winter months. When springtime arrives, the melting effect can have an initial aggravation on fire and water in the body. We may experience congestion, especially if the melting process is blocked in some way. The heaviness of water has accumulated over the winter and begins to melt in spring. Exercises should reflect and assist this process, including more sweating and cleansing programmes at this time of year. Fire imbalances are felt in the lower parts of the body generally and water imbalances are predominantly felt in the upper parts of the body.

Air/Water Types

Air and water both lack heat. Air is light and dry, and water is heavy and moist. Air and water are both cold in nature, though their experience of cold is very different. This lack of heat can manifest as a lack of passion and drive in life. Air/water types can be very laid back, but may allow other, more fiery individuals to dominate them. They need to find strength and passion within themselves. Finding this within will benefit any imbalances in their constitution. Developing heat in an exercise routine and a passion for living can be cultivated. Physically, predominant air and water types are opposite in many ways. Air types are thin and light whereas water types are stocky and heavy. The size and frame of an air/water type would depend on which humour is dominant. They could have a heavy body or a tall and thin body. Fire can be cultivated in order to build up heat and strength as well as the will to exercise routinely.

A lack of fire would show up in the horoscope with the Sun, Mars and the south node weakly placed or not influencing the individual's nature to any great degree. The horoscope would show a challenge for such an individual to express this fiery drive and passion for living. For example, if fire is lacking, it may show that Mars may have little or no influence on the individual's nature. He or she may lack a personal sense of power and ambition in life. Exercises that are heating and more competitive would be more beneficial in this case, perhaps involving them in encouraging team sports.

In the autumn and winter months when air and water dominate in nature, it would be beneficial to follow the natural cycles of things and exercise accordingly. Air dominates in autumn and water in late winter. Even if it is not the season that is representative of the energy you are working with, it is more important to note if you are feeling an increase or decrease of certain energies. Usually when there is a predominance of certain energies, that energy is being accumulated and an excess experienced. It is this excess that causes the imbalance. Although a lack of one of the bodily humours also contributes to an imbalance, it is more usual for an excess to bring about an imbalance as it is easier for a certain type to overdo a humour that is already prominent.

In an air/water constitution, there is a dominance of air and water. These two should be kept balanced in a practice and according to the time of year. With time, awareness of which is imbalanced will guide physical activity depending on how one feels. If there is anxiety present, then use an air approach. If you are feeling heavier and stuck, then a water approach would be beneficial. Similarly, for air/fire types, if they can find a more fluid approach to their routine, it will naturally balance air and fire. This would mean staying with gentler exercises for longer and grounding in the body. Fire/water types could cultivate adaptability in their exercise routine to keep their energy balanced. This would mean being more flexible and offering a more adaptable approach to their routine.

Mixed Types

A mixed type would show all three bodily humours are present in equal proportions in an individual. This may not always be the case and can be, upon closer inspection, observed to be a dual type. If the three are equally present, then all of the energies must be worked with more intimately. This is the case with every one of us, of course, but in this type it becomes even more important. You may think that this is the best type to be and although that might be the case if there is balance, the issue here is to know which of the energies are out of balance when an imbalance is felt.

One thing to remember is that air is the driving force and keeping it in balance will keep the whole system running smoothly. If there is an imbalance, however, it would be advisable to work with all the energies at different times of the day, year and throughout the various stages of life. Working with how each of these energies is felt in different aspects of life can be of great benefit. This will be looked at more closely when we look at Vedic astrology later.

A Golden Rule

When out of balance, we seek things that bring us further out of balance. For an air type, this will be to do too much and becoming edgy and anxious. For a fire type, this will be a need to control things and getting angry when things inevitably do not go a certain way. For a water type, this will be getting stuck and feeling lethargic. When we are in balance, we seek things that keep us in balance. Air types will know they are in balance when they are enthusiastic and creative. Fire types will feel a passion for living and an ability to share their joy of life. Water types will flow gracefully through life while being loving and affectionate. An exercise routine with your constitution in mind can help you gain and maintain balance throughout the day and for all of the years of your life.

The Three Qualities of Each Humour

To understand more of the complexities of each of the humours, we can also see them in relation to each of the three qualities. We are all, of course, complex beings and no matter how much we look at different types, and no matter how intricate the analysis, it is not possible to sum someone up in a type. For the purposes of this book, however, it is useful to become aware of basic types and to work with these, knowing in your own words your own unique nature.

The Qualities of Air

Air can be expressed in terms of a more dull, turbulent or harmonious nature. In other words, air finds an expression through inertia, activity or harmony, depending on certain factors that are observed in the horoscope. When a duller, more inert nature is expressed in an air type, there is fear present which may lead to phobias and activities that further increase this fear. Fear keeps us from experiencing life fully, but it also has the purpose of protecting us from danger. This danger can all too often be in an air type's mind, however, and have no bearing on the reality of a particular situation. This is the influence of the north node, Rahu, which creates irrational fears. Saturn, on the other hand, brings fear of a very real nature that we may need to protect ourselves against.

It is worth remembering that 'like increases like'. If you are in balance, you will seek things that keep you in balance. However, if you are out of balance, you will seek things that bring you further out of balance. This is easily seen in an air type who does too much, not knowing when, or how, to slow down. They can spend their life thinking about the future, inducing fear all the time. What drives them often ends up derailing them. In an air type, when a dull nature is expressed, there is a need to lift out of the sense of fear and get the energy moving once more. When this is achieved, there is a stage of turbulence that an air type finds themselves in for a large portion of their lives. Staying in this state is not possible for long periods of time, however, and eventually there may be a breakdown into exhaustion once more. However, there can be a breakthrough into a more balanced, harmonious quality, although this is not generally achieved after a period of prolonged agitation. It may appear that way on the surface of things as with someone who is exhausted appearing to be at peace. This state of exhaustion is not a balanced state of being, but a state of decay. When air types are in balance, they find themselves being more creative and enthusiastic about life. They know how much energy they have to spend, but they do not spend it all. They enjoy the many changes of life, but appreciate times of tranquillity and calm also. For any of the types, a balanced and harmonious existence is the ultimate goal. Finding your own balance can be undertaken with the aid of physical exercise that suits your type.

When air is expressed through turbulence, there can be an addictive quality to the high one achieves. This high is a false sense of vitality, which sooner or later crashes back down into inertia. If we find ourselves burning the candle at both ends, pushing through exhaustion, creating a false sense of vitality, we eventually exhaust the system. This leads us into a more inert state, which offers us a protective period against further threat. This is often experienced through illness. Fear of further repercussions keeps us from exerting ourselves even more, and even an air type has to slow down and take to the bed.

During the more active stages, air types could also move their energy, enjoying all the thrills and spills that life has to offer, but with the goal in mind of settling down into a more peaceful state afterwards. This state of balance is possible for anyone, at any time. An air type may take longer to settle, but there is lightness to be experienced in such a state, which is, at the same time, a very full experience. This sense of fullness is what air types crave and what drives them to compulsive behaviour in order to try and satisfy this yearning. Addictions, obsessions and compulsions may lead the way to breakthroughs into a peaceful sense of completeness once the extremes of addictions are experienced.

The Qualities of Fire

When fire types find themselves in a more inert space, there can be a need to control and dominate because of fear. This quality of fire may be taken to the extremes and may even result in physical violence. This can be the expression of the warrior-like planet Mars or the irrational south node, Ketu. There is a need to move through the anger and agitation to burn and clear the energy. From this intense, blinding anger, a stage of irritability is reached. This is a more active quality of fire that needs to be moved through in order to reach a more harmonious state of clarity. The stage of activity, which is agitated and turbulent, can be worked with by moving stuck, inert energy outward. Inertia moves down and outward, as opposed to agitation, which moves out and to the sides. This allows for the energy to lift. Once the energy gets moving, ideally it is with the intention of lifting it inward and up into a more balanced state. Fire is expressed at a stage of balance as an illuminating state of being, creating true perception – where all those 'aha' moments are found. After the blinding anger and intense drive forward have subsided, clarity can result.

The difference between the inert and harmonious stages of fire is the difference between the planet Mars and the Sun. Mars creates anger and an ambition to strengthen one's self. The Sun creates clarity and a sense of oneness with everyone and everything and, as a result, will not tolerate anything which is not for the greater good. This is the difference between the burning energy of the toxic state of Mars and the clarifying influence of a strong Sun in the horoscope. In her book *Personal Panchanga and the Five Sources of Light,* Vedic astrologer Komilla Sutton writes: 'The Sun wants to work in accordance with the soul's desires while Mars wants to work according to its individuality, and will therefore be more selfish.'

When a fire type moves into a more turbulent phase, there can be a lot of ambition to be dealt with and to let go of. It is sometimes one of the hardest things for a fire type to do, but when they learn to let go and allow life to just happen, the joy that awaits them is warm and inviting. Otherwise, the intense heat of toxic fire can burn an individual out eventually. When fire types are in balance, they are passionate and joyous beings who allow life to happen, and yet they are able to motivate and inspire others to reach beyond where they currently find themselves. For this reason, fire types make the best fitness instructors. At its best, Mars represents the courage to change what we can and need to change in our lives.

The Qualities of Water

When water types are in an inert space, it is hard for them to see the light at the end of the tunnel. Depression can be the result of this stage. Though it may be hard for them to accept in this state, they need to move through a stage of agitation. This depression is unlike an air- or fire-type depression, where fears of moving or a frustration from failings dominate. In the case of a water-type depression, there is just a feeling of being stuck, with seemingly no way to move forward. This may be balanced in a vigorous exercise regime, but this may also result in an expression of anger that may not be comfortable for them to express. They must move through this stage to find their way to a more balanced and loving state, and not slip back into a darker, duller state. Acceptance and a sense of letting go of old hurts and disappointments are necessary for them to move on and into a more naturally loving space.

Initially, the stagnant stage can be debilitating for water types. Even getting out of bed can be a mammoth task. Once a water type can get moving in some form or another, the slow process of transformation can begin. This may initially be expressed through a slow-start exercise routine. Slow, gentle stretches can gently begin to move the inert energy. Once there is some movement, more dynamic movement can be introduced. Once the energy gets moving, a water type will find that the stores of abundant energy can be accessed. Water types have more stamina than any other type because of this ability to store energy. This may be expressed as an accumulation of fat, for example, but once they realise their staying power, they can be encouraged gently to move through a more agitated stage, ultimately reaching a more peaceful and light stage of harmony. Water is expressed at a stage of balance and harmony as a feeling of love and devotion. They are the most loyal and affectionate of types, so this natural tendency can find a safe home in a more balanced state and, as long as there are no distractions or obstructions in their life, they are usually very loving, contented individuals.

The Ayurvedic View of Exercise

Just as we need to eat a well-balanced meal to achieve health through diet, we also need to be aware of our nature and the impact of a particular diet on our nature. The same can be said of physical activity, where we need to experience the full range of body motion to remain healthy. We also need to be aware of our nature whilst we exercise as this has more of a say on the overall effect of a particular routine than whether a particular exercise is increasing or decreasing a bodily humour. In other words, though each physical activity is seen as either increasing or decreasing for each of the bodily humours, the routine must always be viewed as a whole.

It is of the greatest benefit to know how we can exercise with the awareness of our own unique nature. Learning about each exercise individually, for example, can add logic to an intuitive body movement. However, an awareness of your nature should initially guide the way in which you move. This will help keep you in balance throughout the day, the year and your life. As we engage in our activities with more awareness, we transform them from the mere physical into a vehicle to become more conscious. Structurally, we must be aware of the technicalities of any exercise in order to move safely. This is important when first starting out on a journey of exploration through the body and the body's innate intelligence.

A Suggested Approach for Each Constitution

Using the information already obtained, you could exercise according to your life stage, depending on your constitution and any imbalances that may be felt at any given time. If you feel more anxious, then cultivate an approach that addresses an air imbalance. If you feel you are pushing too hard in life, and tension is a result, then a fire approach may be required. If you feel heavy and lethargic, then a water approach will help to lift your energy. I would encourage you to read all of the guidelines below to become acquainted with how to exercise according to each type, no matter which type you identify with.

Balancing Air

An air type's irregularity must be restrained and yet given full expression in any given exercise. This may be done with a regular routine that includes variations in movement such as dance. Sports may supply this need as long as you do not lose your grounding in the game. Grounding yourself in your own body is always crucial for an air type, and this must be returned to again and again. One way of doing this is by bringing your awareness back into the breath – the connection between the mind and body. Air types need to feel this connection. Awareness of where you are located geographically is also beneficial and starting your day by exercising will prevent any stress from accumulating in your body. The room you exercise in should be kept warm, but not too hot as this might drain your energy. If taking to the outdoors in a cold climate, then make sure you are well covered, especially when it is windy outside. An air type's energy comes in spurts and does not last long so awareness of this is essential. Do not push yourself too hard and be kind to yourself with rests in between more strenuous exercises if this is deemed necessary.

Air types need to feel secure and cared for. Exercise in an encouraging environment that is free from any distractions. If you feel you need the uplifting sounds of music, then allow yourself the comfort of soothing sounds as long as the music is not too loud or aggravating. Use as many props and comforts as you wish, especially in your relaxation afterwards, which is a must for an air type. Always allow for this time in your daily routine. Start your exercise with some vigorous activity, concentrating on building strength and stamina. Anxious energy can be dispelled with an energetic start. However, the goal should be to slow the routine down as you progress. Move in and out of exercises with a sense of fluidity. Try not to develop any jerking movements in whatever form of exercise you choose. Instead, allow the exercise itself to open and undo any build-up of tension over a longer period of time. Give yourself more time to exercise as it may take you more time to undo the tensions that have built up than it will for the other types. However, do not spend all of this time in strenuous activity.

Slow down. This advice would be the same for any of your activities, whether it is brushing your teeth or going about your daily routines. In your exercises, the more you cultivate this slowness, the more this influences your entire life. Have fun to lighten the heart, but move slowly and carefully to ground in your body, feeling fully anything that is asking for attention. Air types love to move, so be aware that if you are out of balance, the tendency will be to do that which imbalances you further. For air types, this is doing too much, too quickly. Air types love to move out of how they are feeling quite often, instead of staying with more uncomfortable emotions. Exercises such as those in hatha yoga are a safe way for you to experience these emotions and move more slowly through them, addressing anything now so that it will not be felt more intensely later. You may also find this expression through dance. Running, especially long distance, will only deplete your already low reserves and, although it will give you the high you crave, it does not necessarily offer you the balance you need.

Exercises such as those in hatha yoga or in t'ai chi are more relaxing forms of exercise, and the most beneficial to the nervous system as well as any irregularity in the mind/body that air types often experience. Air types need this form of exercise more than any other type. This is true for all of us as we get older, as air increases when we age. It is important for everyone to keep the body working smoothly and to help prevent the tendency for structural irregularities. This becomes even more important if you were born an air type. With age, an air type's tendency is to start to become even more nervous and tense in the body and for distortions of the musculoskeletal system to occur. Hatha yoga practices continued into old age will be of great benefit to you in your life.

Balancing Fire

A fire type's need for achievement and perfection in any activity must be facilitated only up to a point. Allow yourself the motivation of getting into a routine, but once there, you should always simply allow it to flow more naturally – opening the body with more awareness. Try not to push into exercises and activities, but instead allow them to gradually open you. Fire types are more prone to injury because of this need to push, whether this is in a yoga practice, in the gym or the great outdoors. Use whatever activity to balance this tendency and get into the habit of not always giving 100 per cent all of the time.

Start your exercise with more vigorous exercises to use up some of the heated energy your type can build up through living life. This increase in heat will increase your need to control. Your *goal* in your activity should be to let go, even if the person beside you in a class environment seems to be doing better than you. Ideally, then you can use this fire energy to motivate yourself and structure a daily routine, but if you feel like your competitive side is winning out, then sometimes exercising alone is helpful. It is when you exercise on your own that you realise there are no competitors, just your own need for achievement and perfection. Exercise in a cool, comfortable room that will not overheat during your routine. Fire types like to exercise outdoors more than any other type – even in the winter – as this keeps their heat in check. Use props even if you do not need them. This will diffuse the tendency to overdo things. Keep the body cool throughout and when performing more strenuous exercises, practise cooling down. Fire types sweat more during exercise due to the predominance of heat in their constitution. In hatha yoga practices, you would normally breathe through the nose unless there is a specific breathing exercise that is utilised through the mouth. A fire type will become aware of the need to breathe through the mouth during strenuous exercises. This is a need to release excess heat, not simply a need for more air. Breathing through the mouth will cool the system down, though the breath is not purified by breathing this way. However, breathing through the nose becomes impossible during some of the types of competitive exercises a fire type likes to engage in. This is just something to be aware of.

Fire types have moderate endurance so exercise more strenuously in the initial stages of your routine with the intention of always letting things happen in their own good time. Slow the exercise down throughout and emphasise a longer cool-down period. If there is an imbalance, then the tendency is to be attracted to those things that bring further imbalance. Observe this and exercise accordingly by keeping cool and holding back a little.

Balancing Water

A water type's resistance must be constantly encouraged towards action and movement in any physical activity. This should be a gradual endeavour, like ice that is gradually thawed. Water types need prodding or they will tend to slow down and stay in activities that facilitate a feeling of ease. Starting an exercise regime is difficult for you, but once started you have the best endurance of any type. Encouraging yourself to start with gentle and passive stretches suits you best, but with the intention of moving into more strenuous exercises as you continue with your routine. Once you have got some energy moving, you can exercise with more vigour. Competitive environments may facilitate this.

Think lightness in your activities and visualise an ease of movement in and out of exercises more swiftly than the other types. This does not mean you should jerk the body as this can cause damage. It may mean needing to move in and out of exercises repeatedly in order to experience more movement in your body. Repeat exercises with shorter holdings, except for more strenuous exercises which could be held for longer periods. This will give you the intense workout you need. The routine should be made up of mostly strenuous exercises that keep motivating the slowness of water into further action and movement. Seated exercises, such as cycling, should be done only to achieve the full range of body movement and balance, but should not be one's sole exercise. Emphasise more strenuous and adaptable exercises that heat and dispel an accumulation of the water humour in the upper parts of the body.

The space in which you exercise should be warm but well ventilated, if you do not exercise outside, to keep the life force moving throughout the body. Only use props if they are needed to exercise safely. Allow your comfort to be the comfort you feel in your well-oiled and resilient body. Relaxation after any exercise should be observed for a short length of time so as not to facilitate the tendency to dose during the day. Whatever exercise you are working with, whether it is difficult for you or not, practise with the intention of lifting the energy so that it can settle into a light, restful state. Water types need continuous motivation so if an instructor is not available to you, you will need to develop consistency in a daily routine. Remind yourself that you have the strength and staying power to see it through. Beginning an exercise is the challenge for your type so give yourself the pat on the back for a job well done after every workout.

The Benefits of Exercise

When air, fire and water are in balance, we increase good health, clarity of mind and build strong immunity. This can easily be observed when we exercise appropriately while keeping a balanced approach in mind. We take in more of the life force through the conscious movement of the breath as we move the body more vigorously. We may increase our ability to perceive things more clearly through exercise, experiencing those 'aha' moments when we are engaged in physical activity. When we feel healthier we make better lifestyle choices that further increase our ability to exercise. This will result in building greater vitality and immunity which then strengthen the aura. We begin to observe our ability to ward off illnesses to a greater extent and feel more grounded in our bodies. These are just some of the benefits of exercise.

The Five Winds

The five winds are the five sub-humours of the air humour. Each governs and controls the life force as well as different bodily functions and mental states at different stages of our interaction with the life force. These winds show how the life force is moving through us while we exercise in a more detailed manner. This will happen regardless of whether there is awareness of this movement, but when you add this awareness, it can help direct the life force where it is needed to create more healing and balance to certain parts of the body.

The Energizing Wind

This wind is primarily located in the head and chest. Breathing exercises as well as meditation increase it. This is the energising wind that governs what we take in through our food, thoughts, impressions and, of course, our breath. Exercises that are inward and forward moving increase it and exercises that are outward will decrease it – as will any type of over-exertion. It is important to note that this wind is active in all the other winds as well, just like air is the governing humour through which fire and water function. This energising wind presides in the head, so Jupiter can be seen to influence this wind by organising all of the other winds in space. Exercising the right amount and in a natural environment will naturally increase the life force as you take in fresh air, good impressions and eat healthy, nutritious food for your constitutional type.

The Upward-Moving Wind

This upward-moving wind is primarily found in the neck. Singing will increase it and is a greater use of this wind than mere speech alone, which will decrease the life force – just as talking too much will deplete your energy. This is an ascending wind that governs our output of energy and the exhalation, speech and will. The planet Saturn relates to this wind and shows the crucial role of our energy output in determining good health. This wind governs expression and the positive energy from our intake of nutritive substances. Exercises that are upward-moving will increase it and ones that are downward will decrease it. Just as it is important to look at how much energy we are taking into the body, it is also important to be aware of the energy we expel. Normally, we expel far too much energy in needless speech, which is best conserved for our exercise routine. You will be aware of this if you continue to talk while exercising. This interrupts the input and output of the breath and, thus, the life force itself, leaving you feeling out of breath.

The Circulating Wind

This wind is found throughout the body. Extending exercises, where the energy is sent out to the periphery, will increase it. This is an expanding wind and governs the outward movement of food, breath, impressions and thoughts. It governs circulation of the physical and mental body. Exercises that are expanding and extending will increase it while exercises that are contracting and centring will decrease it. This wind presides at the sacral region, representing the fluidity in the hips that can become rigid if not kept flexible. Venus and the Moon relate to this wind as the rulers of the water element and our ability to move with fluidity, not just in our bodily movements, but in our lives.

The Equalizing Wind

This wind is found in the navel. Seated exercises will increase it as this is the contracting and centring wind. Its function includes digestions on all levels and maintains our equilibrium. Exercises that increase it are those that contract and centre us, such as sitting postures while exercising. An example of this would be sit-ups. Exercises that decrease it are those that expand the body, such as dance. This wind presides at the solar plexus, giving us the power of digestion and assimilation. This wind can be related to the Sun and the planet Mars, which represent the fire element at the solar plexus.

The Downward-Moving Wind

This wind is found in the lower abdomen. This descending and stabilising wind is responsible for elimination on all levels, as it takes our energy down and grounds us. Exercises that are grounding, such as seated exercises, or strong standing exercises, such as squats, will increase it. The ability to perform a squatting motion will indicate how well this wind operates and, therefore, how well your organs of elimination function. Exercises that are upward-moving will decrease it. This wind presides at the base of the spine; the downward-moving wind relates to our ability to root into the earth while we exercise. Therefore, any strong leg work will give us an awareness of this. The planet Mercury relates to this wind and our ability to root ourselves in the body along with our practical concerns related to the body.

Results of Proper Exercise

There are more subtle benefits to proper exercise beyond the obvious physical improvements we may make. Clarity of mind is the result of a balanced fire through which we digest air, impressions and thoughts. Exercise can bring intelligence and clarity of mind. It brings us to higher states of perception. This is why sometimes when we grapple with an idea, or have a lack of clarity about something, we may exercise and receive the much-needed clarification. Whatever we take in from our environment, we need to be able to digest. The subtle form of fire enables us to assimilate all the energy that is taken in through thoughts and impressions. When it is functioning in the correct manner, we are perceptive. This is reflected in the strength of the Sun in the horoscope and our ability to function with optimal health and well-being. When we exercise, we build a stronger immunity that is the result of balanced water, giving us our mental strength, a feeling of contentedness, patience and concentration. It allows us to ground higher impressions and perceptions. In other words, it allows us to contain the energy we have taken in and assimilated through proper exercise. However, we must be able to transmute the intake of energy or it may dissipate through sexual indulgence. Venus represents the reproductive fluid and is the most refined of the bodily tissues. The reproductive fluid can be cultivated in order to build stronger immunity and vigour. Vigour may be achieved by directing the energy, usually expended in sexual activity, into other activities such as exercise. However, we must also consider that increased well-being can, in turn, increase sexual health, which must be continually cultivated if we are to remain in good health.

To be a healthy individual, we must look beyond just the physical body. When we are increasing the life force, assimilating it and containing it, we are in balance in accordance with higher states of being. Each of these subtle forces needs to be working well for there to be good health. When we begin to exercise, we can look to these energies and understand how they affect us. When we increase physical activity, we are taking in more of the life force by breathing more deeply. However, this must be utilised efficiently so that we can use the energy and its life-giving qualities. The life force does not work alone. We see that none of these subtle energies exists without the other. After taking in more of the life force, we need to be able to digest it and contain what we have digested. The end result is a vigour and immunity that is the subtle result of all the digestive processes working efficiently. Exercise can add to this efficiency.

If, for example, someone is more of an air type and is suffering from low immunity and that person exercises a lot in order to regain health, they are not only further exhausting themselves through physical activity, but they are also taking in more air with increased respiration. They may lack the ability to digest the increased amount of energy input and may not be able to contain it as a result. In fact, as there is little containment in an air type who is out of balance, there is little protection and the nervous system can be put under duress. It is important to see these subtle energies and how they work in such an instance. This is an example of why too many intense breathing exercises can over-stimulate and ultimately imbalance an air type. Air types must make sure they have enough endurance for lots of exercises that naturally increase their intake of air. They need to make sure they have built up enough immunity and insulation for such exercises through proper, well-balanced lifestyle habits, and at least some retention of the sexual fluids.

Similarly, an individual who builds up immunity through sexual abstinence and lifestyle habits needs to be able to transform this accumulated energy through sufficient exercise. Otherwise it may accumulate, leaving a feeling of heaviness. This is usually the experience of a water type. This is like an overprotective influence that can lead to a feeling of suffocation. More exercises and heat may be required in such a case.

Building healthy bodies by balancing the three bodily humours of air, fire and water, according to each individual's unique ratio of these three, will ultimately lead to a healthy expression by building strong immunity. Living a healthy lifestyle in accordance with your type will be of the utmost importance in achieving this objective. You were born a certain type and that does not change. You are seeking to become in balance with your true nature and constitution, even though this is seen as the universe expressing an imbalance in the greater scheme of things. By adhering to your unique nature, and a balance that is unique to you, you can build great immunity and strength through your exercise routine.

CHAPTER 3 - TIMELINES

Life Stages

The water humour is dominant in the early, formative part of life when we build up our body's mass. Our bodies have a higher percentage of water when younger. The fire humour is dominant in the middle part of life from adolescence onwards when our outward drive and ambition come into play. The air humour is dominant in the later stage of life when our bodies start to lose their flexibility and mass as old age sets in with a drying effect taking place. We have less percentage of water when we age so this must be considered when exercising, and allowances need to be made when there is less lubrication as a result.

Natural Planetary Cycles

The natural cycles of our lives according to planetary influence and dominance begin with the first year of life and the Moon's influence. It is in this formative year of life that we bond with the mother (or not) and this has a profound effect on our entire experience of life. The next two years are governed by Mars up to the age of three, and it is here that we develop our individual needs separate to our mother as we begin to express our individuality. Mercury governs the period of life from the age of three until twelve years of age. This is when we learn most of what we have to learn in life that carries us through this life experience in a practical manner. Venus governs the period of life from twelve until thirty-two. It is at this stage that we initially experience puberty and subsequently develop relationships beyond this into adulthood. The Jupiter period is from the ages of thirty-two until fifty. This period is concerned with the household, raising children and pursuing the things one loves to create. After the age of fifty until the age of seventy-four, we experience our golden years, which is represented by the Sun. The last stage of our life, after the age of seventy-four until we die, is represented by Saturn, as we begin to recede from life.

These are the natural time cycles in all of our lives and we each experience them uniquely, depending on our experience of each of these planets – according to their strength and position in our horoscopes. We also experience planetary periods that are calculated for each horoscope. While many of these planetary periods are calculated based on the specific horoscope, the one dealing with possible current imbalances is relevant for everyone. We will examine this issue in the last chapter (Chapter 7: Changing Patterns).

Seasons

The air humour accumulates in summer and is aggravated in autumn and early winter. During the autumn, the drying effect in nature aggravates air and those of an air-dominant constitution will feel this more than other types. This will express itself as rigidity in the body and emotions, as the cold winds begin to distort the body into uncomfortable shapes, not allowing emotions to move through the body as easily. The body can hunch over in order to keep warm in the colder months and we feel the effect of this on a mental/emotional level, not just in the physical body. Heat will relieve such conditions, but moisture is needed also. Oiling the body with warm oils at this time of year will relieve much of this aggravation. Staying wrapped up and warm, especially when it is cold and windy outside, will help to address the increase of dryness in nature. Follow the balancing air guidelines explained in Chapter 2 in order to address any imbalances, especially if you are an air type.

The fire humour accumulates in spring and is aggravated in the summer. The summer months can aggravate a fire type by overheating them and making them impatient and angry. Whether this anger is expressed outwardly or not is another matter. This heat can lead to all kinds of inflammatory conditions. Cooling down with cooling oils and meditation will help alleviate these conditions, as will laughter, which can relieve the stressful build-up of heat.

The water humour accumulates in winter and is aggravated in the spring. This increases phlegmatic conditions over the winter months, and once spring comes along, the build-up of heaviness and coldness begins to melt as it meets with the heat of summer. This heating is initially aggravating to the water humour and is observable in springtime in many suffering from all kinds of congestive disorders. This is also because we react to the cold of winter by storing up on heavy, comforting foods at that time of year. In order to address this in a daily routine, you could exercise with balancing water in mind – accentuating cleanses in order to allow the excess water to move up and out. Excesses of the water humour need to move up to move out as these excesses are felt mostly in the upper part of the body in the stomach, chest, throat and head. An excess of air and fire needs to be released by moving it down and out. This can be achieved through cleansing the lower parts of the body.

Time of Day

The fire humour is related to the day and is more prominent at noon and midnight. The water humour is related to the night and the hours before midday and midnight. The air humour is related to the transitions between day and night, i.e., dusk and dawn.

	Day	Night
Water	7am-11am	7pm-11pm
Fire	11am-3pm	11pm-3am
Air	3pm-7pm	3am-7am

Planetary Divisions of the Day

The Sun rules the day and the Moon rules the night. Although this might seem obvious due to the Sun's prominence during the day and the Moon's prominence at night, certain approaches to living – when certain lifestyles are taken into account – can leave some out of synch within these natural cycles. This out of synch approach is apart from the fact that many are more productive at different times of the day. This pattern of productivity will be reflected in each individual's unique nature. Air and fire types find it easier to get going first thing in the morning if they are in balance. Water types find it challenging to start the day with any great enthusiasm, but have more endurance throughout the day if they are in balance. There is a natural sense for all of us in how best to approach life on a daily basis. Metabolism is divided into solar and lunar phases each day as catabolic hormones break down molecules in order to release energy during the day and anabolic hormones build molecules at night in order to repair the body after the exertions of the day.

The Planets and the Days of the Week

Each planet rules a day of the week. Sunday is the Sun's day, Monday the Moon's day, Tuesday is Mars' day, Wednesday is Mercury's day, Thursday is Jupiter's day, Friday is Venus' day and Saturday is Saturn's day. Pay attention to each of the planets on its day of the week by approaching activities and exercises accordingly as well as performing activities which are conducive to that planet.

Sunday

On Sundays, you may wish to perform activities with a sense of honouring your Higher Self. Traditionally for many, it is the day to visit a place of worship, but if this is not for you, then you may also create a space for yourself at home. Making your space a more uplifting experience can be of great benefit, remembering that whatever you may worship is a reflection of the spirit within you. Spending some time in meditation will help to deepen this connection to your Higher Self. If it is sunny outside, then make sure to allow the light to shine into your space. Getting some of the Sun's rays will, of course, give you more of a sense of this connection.

If you decide to exercise on this day, you could use some rhythmic music and drumming in your workout. The Sun was always worshipped by ancient people by beating a drum. This is because the Sun is very rhythmic in its movement, moving one degree through the zodiac each day, giving us a sense of time through the seasons of the year. You may wish to pay more attention to the rhythm of your life and your exercise programme on this day. If you practise yoga, then you may wish to pay particular attention to the Sun salutations. Watch how the light moves across the room, highlighting different parts of your space. If it is possible to feel the heat of the Sun on your body, then do so, knowing that you are a spark from our one source of light.

Monday

On Mondays, you may wish to meditate or spend some time being more contemplative. Resting your awareness at the heart will take you out of your head space and access the stillness of your being. The more time you spend at the heart, the more you can access a deeper awareness of self, beyond the mind's commentary. Spending time by the water, or simply taking a bath, will help bring you into more of a connection to nature and the water element. Learning to work with the waxing and waning phases of the Moon will help this process as you learn to go with the flow of the natural world. During the new Moon phases, it is best to remain quiet and contemplative as the previous two weeks of the waning Moon have been a time of letting go. The full Moon allows for more energy and expression, but is also a good time to step back a bit from too much activity, since the previous two weeks of the waxing phase have gradually increased our worldly concerns. This would apply to any physical activity also. Exercise with caution during a full Moon and a new Moon as the high energy of a full Moon can lead to injury and the low energy of a new Moon can deplete you even further if you over-extend yourself.

Tuesday

On Tuesdays, you may wish to be more active and express yourself more physically and competitively. This is a good day to take on a task that you have been putting off. Use the courage of Mars to tackle something uncomfortable in your life. Although this is not an auspicious day for new beginnings, if there is a situation where you need to tackle something you need to improve or completely remove from your life, then this would be a good day for it. Make sure to keep the toxic heat of Mars at bay by exercising in a way that allows the heat to be utilised and then released if needed. Exercise with courage and conviction, knowing that any discomfort you feel can help balance your tendency to luxuriate in an imbalanced state. Sometimes we have to do things that do not feel good to us, but they are necessary if we wish to destroy those things that keep us feeling weak or held back in some way.

Wednesday

On Wednesdays, you may wish to learn something new or how to work more analytically with something you already know. If there is a need for stimulation of the mind, it would be best facilitated by studying something of value to you in your life or by engaging with others in team sports. Mercury represents the earth element, which corresponds to our very practical concerns. You may wish to use this day to deal with the practicalities of your life, which on other days may seem too trivial or tedious.

Thursday

On Thursdays, you may wish to follow a teacher or teachings that broaden your horizons in some way. This could be expanded upon to include anyone in your life who has something to teach you. You could also seek out a place you have never been before in order to expand your world view. Observe the beliefs you hold and how they serve you on your life journey. Tune into your 'inner voice' and know that you always have access to this guidance. You may wish to access this through listening to the sounds in your environment initially, before settling on the silence that is ever-present. Explore the space between the breaths as you dive deeper into a feeling of inner space and the innate intelligence of your body.

Friday

On Fridays, you may wish to relax and be at ease in your body. This is a good day to experience happiness and contentment in whatever form this comes in for you. In exercise, you may wish to enjoy your body more on this day. Feel the fluidity of your body through dance if you enjoy this type of exercise. Find what makes you happy and gives you a sense of contentment, and enjoy it today. However, instead of overindulging – which you will only have to work harder at paying for tomorrow – you may simply observe the ability to be happy without needing something to give you that feeling. There is no need for more things, situations, people or places to be present for you to feel content with what is right now. Enjoy simply being you and the pleasure your body gives you.

Saturday

Saturday is the best day for clearing any excesses brought about in the week. This may be through a food fast or mentally fasting with the aid of meditation. Saturday is the best day to clear out the excesses and to do chores around the house as well as cleaning our bodies out through some form of cleansing. Use this day to appease Saturn and suffer voluntarily! However, you should only perform a fast after you have consulted a healthcare professional. If you are currently experiencing sadness in your life, then you are appeasing an energy that is alive in you and is looking for expression. In suffering voluntarily by limiting the amount you indulge in, you purposefully invite the limitations of Saturn into your day and, in doing so, you may not have to experience as much of the negative expressions of the planet of restrictions, delays and obstructions. Fasting allows you to experience these with a light touch and a clear mind. You can view your life more objectively and with more detachment. While you fast, you are detoxifying the body and clearing the mind to lighten up and refresh yourself for the week ahead.

For those who need to keep an adequate amount of nutrients, a juice fast (though strictly not a fast) may be an alternative to a complete fast, although you would ideally use appropriate juices for your constitutional type. Failing that, a half-fast may be observed. This may mean consuming light foods throughout the day or having a simple meal in the evening, avoiding heavy and stimulating foods throughout the day. The objective is to give something up that can benefit your mind and body, not denying yourself that which you need to remain physically healthy. Most people eat excessively and benefit from a one-day fast per week. However, if you are an air type and are experiencing an aggravation of air, leading to further weight loss, it may not be advisable to observe a food fast. In such a case, a day of silence or giving something up you would normally indulge in during the rest of the week may be better approaches.

CHAPTER 4 – AYURVEDIC ASTROLOGY

The Vedic horoscope represents our nature on every level of our being. Although the science of astrology is more subtle than the influence of our environment on Earth, the influence of the planets has a more powerful effect on us because of their subtlety. If you are aware of the effect an environment, a food substance or a situation has on your being, then you can acknowledge and work with it more consciously. If, however, the influence is so subtle that you are not conscious of it, there is a need to become more conscious in order to live life more skilfully. The influence of the planets is no different to what an Ayurvedic doctor would point out in an examination or through your own awareness brought about by any means. We can, however, through an awareness of the movement of the planets, bring this to a more conscious awareness and work with these influences within time frames and patterns that are easily identifiable in the Vedic horoscope. Astrology is all about timing, whether it is timing an appropriate exercise or how best to approach such an activity at any given time.

The nine 'planets' studied in Vedic astrology are known as the nine *Grahas* or 'seizers'. The Sanskrit word *Graha* means 'to grab' or 'to grasp'. This shows how the planets can take hold of us and express themselves in our lives, making sure we are directed to live out the results of previous thoughts, words and actions. If we are more influenced by a certain planet from birth, then we will express its qualities more than the others. We will, however, express all of the planets in some way, as each area of our life experiences different results. Here, the notion of an individual being more influenced by a certain quality overall is in relation to their rising sign in the horoscope and the planets influencing this sign.

The planets influence us on every level of our being and express their qualities through us. If we are more influenced by the planet Saturn, for example, then we are more influenced by inertia and reflect this in our nature. Though we can reach beyond this earthly experience, and touch into our pure being, we still must adhere to the laws of the universe while we are in a physical body. We need to work with them more effectively if we wish to manage our lives more skilfully. We also express the qualities of particular planets more during certain times of our life, depending on what period we are currently experiencing and where that planet is transiting through our horoscope. This will show where the planet's quality is focused at any particular time. A period of a particular planet will express not only its influence due to its inherent nature, but its influences based on its more specific role for each individual as seen in its placement at birth. It also influences us as it moves around the horoscope by transit, i.e., the different areas of our life. In this way it can be seen that the 'planet', or *graha*, has a hold of us and it then becomes a skill in working with these influences every day with a healthy approach to each of the planets. The planets are a representation of various aspects of our being. When we understand this, we can make friends with any circumstance or impulses we experience at any given time. In time, we can learn how to make the most of every influence while fully accepting its quality in our life.

The best way to understand how the planets influence us is to study the effects of the three qualities (activity, harmony and inertia), which in turn give us the five elements (space, air, fire, water and earth) and result in the three bodily humours (air, fire and water). The three qualities operate on a psychological level more than the humours, though they influence each other. Our minds can be seen to change according to the influences of the three qualities more rapidly than our bodies. Our bodies do change, of course, though not as rapidly as our minds. We have a sense of them being more solid and static, although they are impulses that change more slowly. Our minds affect the state of our bodies and vice versa. When we look at our physical body, we can see it is remaining somewhat stable. We are born with some physical characteristics that have not seemed to have changed in the course of our lives, although we know that is not true and that every cell in our bodies is continually changing – giving us a completely new body every few years. It is, however, changing within similar patterns. This gives us a sense of our nature as seen in the three biological humours of Ayurveda. However, this is not the full picture, so a study of the qualities and elements is required, which can be seen in the reflection of the planets.

The Nine Heavenly Bodies

The Sanskrit word *Graha* encompasses all the visible heavenly bodies and the two calculated nodes of the Moon or eclipse points. They are:

The luminaries – The Sun and the Moon.

The five planets – Mercury, Venus, Mars, Jupiter and Saturn.

The lunar nodes – *Rahu,* the north node, and *Ketu,* the south node.

The Nature of Each Planet

Just as we have our nature, which is a complex and intricate thing, the planets have their inherent nature (for ease in reading I refer to the *Grahas* as planets). Our own complexities are seen in the unique planetary configuration at the time of birth. The planets have their inherent qualities, which are modified depending on where they are placed at any given time. They do not stand apart from anything else, but are influenced by them – just as we do not stand alone without influence from others and our environment. The following is a brief description of the nature of each of the planets. We will look at each in more detail in the next chapter.

The Sun

The Sun represents fire in a harmonious state if well placed in the horoscope. This represents a person with robust health. That is to say, it is fiery in nature, but it is a fire that brings about true perception and vitality, burning away any impurities. Just as a little Sun is detoxifying, we can benefit from the Sun when it is taken with due respect.

The Moon

The waning and new Moon are 'airy' in nature and the waxing and full Moon are 'watery' in nature. The Moon shows mental and emotional health. A well-placed Moon is also harmonious along with the Sun and these two luminaries show the Self (Sun) and the projected mind and emotions (Moon). Just as the Moon reflects the light of the Sun and has no light of its own, our minds reflect our own reality that is our own personal perspective. We see our world through our own lens and experience life through the senses. This is represented by the Moon in the horoscope. This world view is marked by our likes and dislikes, and is a very personal experience. The influences on the Moon itself will show one's mental and emotional nature and which of the qualities are dominating at any given time in an individual's psychological makeup.

Mars

Mars represents fire, which can cause disease through excess heat and toxins. The Sun is more harmonious, bringing about a purifying effect, and Mars represents our selfish needs, which create difficulty for others. Mars also represents the harm we cause to ourselves by protecting our own self-interests, but it can also show the very necessary protection we are afforded in some situations, such as self-defence. The Sun can be seen as Self-centred whereas Mars is selfish. Mars represents the need to do something with what we perceive will strengthen us or to destroy something that weakens us, whether mentally, emotionally or physically.

Mercury

Mercury represents the intellect. It shows our ability to separate ourselves from an emotional involvement in order to view something rationally. Mercury is seen as having the attributes of all three humours. It is more active in nature, being the fastest-moving planet (not including our Moon). It takes on the attributes of the other planets it associates with. In this way, we see that our mind is very easily influenced by what we feed it. We can see the active nature of Mercury in our minds, which are easily agitated and always looking for external stimuli.

Jupiter

Jupiter represents a 'watery' nature, although it corresponds to space. This is because space contains all of the elements and has a binding quality, which gathers the elements and creates a larger body type, i.e., a water-type body. Water is the container of the body's structure and maintains harmony. Jupiter corresponds to our inner intelligence as opposed to Mercury, which corresponds to the intellect. This deeper intelligence does not need external data to process information, but instead arrives at its intelligence through an internal and spontaneous process.

Venus

Venus is active like Mercury. It shows our need to always seek things that are pleasurable as we experience life through the senses. It has both an 'airy' and a 'watery' nature – gathering and dispersing the tissues in a pleasing manner that is reflected in a voluptuous body. As with all of the planets, this will be greatly affected by its sign position and interaction with other planets. While Mars represents our needs that fulfil our selfish desires – the 'fire in our belly' – Venus represents our willingness to compromise in order to suit another. It sensitises us to our environment and to those around us. This is reflected in the amount of flexibility we obtain in the body.

Saturn

Saturn is inert in nature and the primary representation of air. It is the planet that causes most diseases as the air humour has the most classifications for disease in the science of Ayurveda. Saturn shows where we must experience our greatest challenge to our health – physically, mentally and emotionally. It brings a sense of separation into our lives and is a stage at which we need to develop detachment. Venus and the Moon make us aware of others and their needs, but Saturn asks us to withdraw to consider our own limitations in this space and time.

Rahu – The Moon's North Node

The north node is dark and 'airy' in nature. It can be seen as Saturn's alter ego. Whereas Saturn represents air, resulting in negative thinking and bad habits if poorly placed in the horoscope, the north node represents a disturbance to the air element and the resulting chaos brought about by irrational thinking. The north node and Saturn are both similar in many ways, having the predominance of air in their makeup. However, where Saturn represents real fears, the north node represents irrational fears and is experienced psychologically. They both rule the air-dominant sign Aquarius.

Ketu – The Moon's South Node

The south node is toxic and fiery in nature. It is similar to Mars in that respect. They both rule the same sign of the zodiac, Scorpio. The south node, just like the north, causes psychological disturbances and can be seen as an intensified Mars impulse in many ways. If Mars is a fire burning away anything that is perceived to weaken us, the south node is a laser beam cutting through our worldly experience entirely. This allows us to go beyond this material existence. Disillusionment with this worldly experience results from the south node's influence.

General Planetary Indications

The inert, dull and toxic planets – Saturn, Mars and the nodes – cause more illnesses, though any planet can cause illness depending on the strength and position in the horoscope. Even the most benevolent planet Jupiter can cause illness, as seen when placed in the 1st house, which can cause too much weight and lead to obesity. This is because Jupiter is not only 'watery' in nature, but also the largest planet in our solar system as well as representing the adipose (fat) tissue in the body. If you are more influenced by a planet that is more toxic in nature, either inherently or periodically, then you are influenced by more selfishness and self-serving impulses. Mars brings a selfish desire to achieve something for ourselves in order to find strength. Saturn gives us a sense of our separate self and protects our self-interests by holding us back in fear. The nodes of the Moon bring a more distorted view of reality and of the self as they eclipse the Sun and the Moon, representing our true self and projected self.

If we are more influenced by the more active planets Venus and Mercury, we will display a more goal-oriented, yet inclusive nature. This would show a selfish need, but with the ability to include others in those selfish desires. Balance and harmony are possible with the Sun and Moon as well as the planet Jupiter, if they are well placed in the horoscope. If we are more influenced by these celestial bodies, we will display more altruistic pursuits in life or, at the very least, altruistic pursuits may be more pronounced during their time periods.

Conception

Your mother and father's nature came together to create life at the moment of your conception. The result of this blending is seen at the time of your birth and this is reflected in your Vedic horoscope. Astrology is all about timing, so if you do not know your time of birth, you will need to consult a Vedic astrologer who will be able to rectify your chart to arrive at a correct time of birth for you. If you have already obtained your Vedic horoscope, you should be able to ascertain the positions of the Sun and Moon, the five planets and the nodes of the Moon (Rahu and Ketu) in your horoscope. You should also be able to ascertain your rising sign. For a correct calculation, you will need to be working with an *exact* time of birth, which is usually obtained from hospital records if a parent is not present or does not have the time recorded.

Body, Mind & Soul

You can still use the following information even if you do not know your exact time of birth. You may choose to work with your Moon sign as a starting point instead, which may be obtained from knowing only an approximate birth time. Failing that, you may begin to work with your Sun sign. However, the rising sign is most useful when wishing to understand your constitution and body. Each of these three calculated points represents a starting point in the interpretation of your horoscope. The slowest to change is the Sun, which moves signs in the middle of each month in the sidereal zodiac used in Vedic astrology. The fastest to move is the rising sign, with a different sign rising on the eastern horizon approximately every two hours. The Moon changes signs every two and a half days approximately, which should be easy to calculate for most – unless the time is not known and the Moon may appear to move signs within the birth date given. These three calculated points in your horoscope represent your body (rising sign), mind (Moon) and soul (Sun). If you have your chart and notice a gathering of planets in a particular sign, then you may look to that sign and its nature also in order to see more of your own nature. Nothing is viewed in isolation. So, even if you know your rising sign, it is still viewed within the context of the entire horoscope.

Constitution in the Horoscope

To begin the study of your unique constitution, as expressed in the Vedic horoscope, the first thing to examine is the *Lagna* or 'rising sign'. This is the sign that was rising (ascending) on the eastern horizon when you were born. It is also known as the ascendant. The Sanskrit word *Lagna* is often translated as 'marriage', which represents the marriage between heaven and earth on the eastern horizon. It represents the space captured on the eastern horizon as the skies met the earth, encapsulating you in your physical body as you emerged from your mother's womb.

There are many things to examine in the horoscope to arrive at a conclusion as to a person's constitution and any imbalances being experienced at any given time. This would involve a static analysis for a constitutional type and a combination of a static and dynamic analysis for any imbalances. I have kept this analysis as simple as possible – leaving out many of the elements that can be studied in order to come to a more accurate interpretation – as they would only create confusion at this point. I have remained mostly within the realms of a static analysis, which does not take into account current transits, although I have included a planetary period analysis to some degree in the last chapter of this book. My intention with this is to inspire you to delve deeper if the need arises at some point, not to put you off further study. Taking a look at the most basic of indications of health and constitution in the horoscope, we must first look to the rising sign and its ruling planet. Your nature is strongly influenced by this and, as we will examine later, the rising sign in the 9th divisional chart. Planets that are strongly placed also have an impact on your nature. The planet that rules your rising sign plays the most important role in your overall health and will be studied more in-depth in the following chapter. For now, let us look at some of the required areas of study to ascertain your constitution.

Some Things to Examine Constitution:

- The dominant element of your rising sign and its ruling planet, as well as the nature of the sign itself.
- Any planets placed in, or influencing, your rising sign.
- The position of the sign's ruling planet as well as the planets that influence this planet.
- The four angular houses in the chart. These are the 4th, 7th and 10th houses along with the 1st house or rising sign.
- Strongly positioned planets.

Table of Planets

Planet	Quality	Humour	Sign(s) ruled
Sun	Harmonious	Fire	Leo
Moon	Harmonious	Air and Water	Cancer
Mars (Fire)	Inert	Fire	Aries and Scorpio
Mercury (Earth)	Active	Mixed	Gemini and Virgo
Jupiter (Space)	Harmonious	Water	Sagittarius and Pisces
Venus (Water)	Active	Air and Water	Taurus and Libra
Saturn (Air)	Inert	Air	Capricorn and Aquarius
Rahu	Inert	Air	Aquarius
Ketu	Inert	Fire	Scorpio

Planetary Relationships

One way to ascertain the strengths and weaknesses of a planet, and that elemental force within, is to see if the planet is placed in a friendly or unfriendly environment. The planets interact with each other in some way or another, although some are more cooperative than others. The planet Jupiter rules the fire-dominant sign Sagittarius and the water-dominant sign Pisces. This makes the planet friendly towards the Sun and Moon, both of which represent these elements. Mars also rules a fire-dominant and water-dominant sign, i.e., Aries and Scorpio, and makes it conducive to the workings of the Sun and Moon. If you think of the Sun and Moon as royalty, the Sun being the King and the Moon, the Queen, then you can understand the relationship that Jupiter and Mars have to the throne. Jupiter is the advisor and Mars the commander of the kingdom's armies. Both of these work with and alongside the King and Queen.

Mercury rules Gemini and Virgo, Venus rules Taurus and Libra, and Saturn rules Capricorn and Aquarius. Because all of these signs are air- and earth-dominant, these planets are friendly towards each other. One way to observe this friendship is by looking at the beauty of Venus being expressed through the structure of Saturn in a framed painting and the business of selling such a painting in the marketplace (Mercury). There are also planetary relationships that are neutral due to the intricacies of their individual relationships.

Planet	Friends	Enemies	Neutral
Sun	Moon, Mars, Jupiter	Saturn, Venus	Mercury
Moon	Sun, Mercury	None	All others
Mars	Sun, Moon, Jupiter	Mercury	Venus, Saturn
Mercury	Sun, Venus	Moon	Mars, Jupiter, Saturn
Jupiter	Sun, Moon, Mars	Mercury	Saturn
Venus	Mercury, Saturn	Sun, Moon	Mars, Jupiter
Saturn	Mercury, Venus	Sun, Moon, Mars	Jupiter

Strengths and Weaknesses

Planetary strengths and weaknesses are a complex study, using many different criteria to analyse the overall strength of a planet. To begin, you may simply look at the table on page 66 to get a very general indication of whether a planet is strongly or weakly placed in your horoscope. These positions are always modified greatly by other indications. You may also take note of whether a planet is placed in a friendly or unfriendly environment based on the previous table of planetary friendships. For now, you may wish to take note of any planetary positions you have in the signs listed. You may compare how these planets are placed in the main birth chart and the 9th divisional chart, which sits alongside your main chart. This should be provided by a reputable Vedic astrologer or Vedic astrology resource.

If you see a planet is debilitated in the main chart (see the following table on Planetary Strengths), but exalted in the 9th divisional chart, then that is a very different picture, and one which paints a more accurate portrait of the strength of that planet. In that case, the planet would find a great strength that is more often hidden and may not find as easy an expression in the outer world – yet one that is there nonetheless. Similarly, if a planet is exalted in the main chart and debilitated in the 9th division, there may be strength afforded that area of your life in the outer world, yet is one that feels like a weakness on a deeper level of your being. Look to see how well placed each planet is by its position in the main chart versus the position in the 9th divisional chart. If a planet is placed in the same sign in the main horoscope and in the 9th divisional chart, then that indicates strength for that planet no matter which sign it may be. Of course, if it were placed in exaltation in both charts, then this would indicate a great strength.

Just as the Moon waxes and wanes, we can see the planets growing in strength as they move from debilitation to exaltation and lessening their strength as they move from exaltation to debilitation. Although exact degrees are listed in the table given, you can also view the planets' placement in the sign referred to as a whole. A whole sign consists of 30 degrees. The placement of a planet will either strengthen or weaken the indications of that planet depending on whether the planet is closer to the exact degree or having moved past that degree. When considering degrees, always be aware if a planet is at a very low degree or very high degree in a sign. This means it has either just entered the sign or is about to leave. The planet loses strength in this instance, just as you would lose strength by moving house!

Firstly, take note of the planet that rules your rising sign. This is given in the table of the signs of the zodiac. Then look to see its position in your chart in relation to the degrees in the table. Is the planet moving to or from its point of exaltation/debilitation?

Planetary Strength

	Exaltation	**Debilitation**	**Trinal Strength**
Sun	10° Aries	10° Libra	Leo 0 – 20°
Moon	3° Taurus	3° Scorpio	Taurus 4 – 30°
Mars	28° Capricorn	28° Cancer	Aries 0 – 12°
Mercury	15° Virgo	15° Pisces	Virgo 16 – 20°
Jupiter	5° Cancer	5° Capricorn	Sagittarius 0 – 10°
Venus	27° Pisces	27° Virgo	Libra 0 – 15°
Saturn	20° Libra	20° Aries	Aquarius 0 – 20°

Trinal Strength

There is a special placement for each planet in which there is a great strength afforded the planet. This is known as *Moolatrikona* or 'trinal strength' and is included in the above table. This is a very effective position for any planet and one that guarantees a strong expression for the planet. Although a planet may be placed in exaltation, this may be cancelled due to other factors as well as the fact that having a particular malevolent planet strongly placed may not always be a beneficial experience. In most cases, having an exalted planet reveals great expectations in that area of life which may lead to disappointments. In some cases, having a planet in debilitation is actually preferable. In other cases, having a planet in debilitation can indicate a planet that is unable to express its nature or, in the case of malevolent planets, an even more malevolent expression may be found. Please do not take your planet in exaltation or debilitation as simply 'good' or 'bad'. It is a telling position, as everything is, but you must decide on the overall result of this for yourself.

Here are some questions to ask yourself in relation to the strength of each of the planets in your own chart. Have you found meaning (strength of Jupiter) in life, beyond a sense of pleasure and happiness (strength of Venus), and a sense of discipline and courage (strength of Mars), as you deal with your life responsibility and with a loving detachment (strength of Saturn)? Have you been able to develop skills that have served you in living in the material world (strength of Mercury), while balancing these more rational concerns with a healthy emotional life (strength of the Moon)? Have you a sense of identity and are able to express your soul's purpose confidently (strength of the Sun), while finding new ways to live, as you evolve (strength of *Rahu*) beyond where you have a sense of coming from (strength of *Ketu*)? These are just a few examples of how the planets find a strong expression in our life experience.

Examining Constitution

To begin an exploration into your constitution at birth, we will look at the 1st house as this relates to your physical body, and we can relate this to your exercises more easily. However, nothing is viewed in isolation so I need to make some general statements, which I hope you apply to your own awareness as a means to enhance your understanding. You could apply this to your Moon sign in order to see the psychological impact, or your Sun sign and your experience of a Higher Self and identity. These three points in the horoscope represent body, mind and soul. Although they do not tell the whole story, they are a good place to start.

You may also wish to look at the position of all of the five planets – Jupiter, Saturn, Mars, Venus and Mercury – in order to see how you experience each of the corresponding elements of space, air, fire, water and earth. By counting all of the planets in each sign, you will see which elements are dominant. You may wish to read the section on the elements again with this new-found awareness. Remember that all of the planets have their own nature, although this is modified by sign placement and their interaction with other planets. To begin, you may just take note of the position of planets by sign placement in your chart.

If, for example, you wish to view the strength of your Sun in the chart – the Sun representing the fire humour – it is balanced fire if well placed. If your Sun were placed in the sign Aries, it would add a more 'fiery' quality to the Sun. This may play out in a person's life through a strong sense of self and may burn those who stand in the way of their purpose and identity. If Mars were in a strong position, then the burning would be more severe on others as Mars represents that part of us that is not concerned for others. The Sun will burn you eventually, but it will give you plenty of time and warning before such a burning takes place as well as there being benefit from the heat in the meantime.

If you have ever stood in the presence of an individual with a very strong identity, you will no doubt enjoy the heat from such a passionate soul – that is until you try and impinge on their sense of self and purpose for being.

The Houses of Astrology

House	Some Significations	Indicative of ...	Body part
1	Self, nature, confidence	Sun	Head/body
2	Food, resources, family	Jupiter	Face/mouth
3	Younger siblings, courage	Mars	Upper chest/arms
4	Home, mother, comforts	Venus/Moon	Chest/heart
5	Creativity, children, mantra	Jupiter	Heart/Solar Plexus
6	Enemies, disease, bad habits	Saturn/Mars	Lower abdomen
7	Relationships, marriage	Venus	Pelvic region
8	Debts, secrets, inheritance	Saturn	Genitalia/anus
9	Father, advisors, beliefs	Jupiter	Hips & thighs
10	Career, status, karma	Mercury/Sun/Mars	Knees
11	Friends, gains, older siblings	Jupiter	Legs
12	Loss, forgiveness	Saturn	Feet

Cosmic Man

In the table of the houses, you will notice how each house represents a part of the body just as each sign of the zodiac represents a part of the body. In this way, we can see the natural order from Aries to Pisces, representing the body from head to toe. This way of viewing the zodiac is known as the *Kalapurusha* or 'cosmic man', the notion of man mapped out in the zodiacal belt representing the various parts of the body – limited by the experience of time (*Kala*). This can be used in more specific analysis, but for now we will concentrate on the 1st house, which represents the body overall. A strongly placed planet will indicate strength for the body part which that planet represents in your horoscope. A weakly placed planet will indicate an inherent weakness for that body part. Refer to the table of houses and table of planetary strengths, taking note of any planets you may have in debilitation. Look to see which body parts this debilitated planet corresponds to by counting inclusively from your rising sign to the sign this planet rules in your horoscope Then take the house position of this sign to see which corresponding body part is affected.

If you have obtained your birth chart data and know the positions of the rising sign, Moon and Sun, then you may begin to observe how your body, mind and spirit are placed using the tables given. You may wish to further investigate by observing the positions of the planets, but at this point it is enough to just work out the positions and become familiar with some of the signs' attributes. We will build upon this subsequently in order to give you a more in-depth look at each planet and sign.

Once a house position is known, the analysis is no longer only general and can be personalised for you. Once you know your rising sign, you can then personalise all of the planets, according to what they represent for you specifically, and where they are located in your horoscope. This will show where they have more of an influence by position, and by the areas of life they have an influence on, i.e., the houses they rule in your horoscope as well as the aspects they cast as they influence different areas of your life (we will look at aspects later).

For the purposes of this book, we will focus on the first house, representing the body and the constitution. This needs to be looked at in relation to the influences upon it.

In Fig. 1, I have given the layout of the signs of the zodiac in the south Indian-style chart layout. In this chart layout, the signs of the zodiac remain in the same positions as the rising sign moves position. So, for example, if you have the sign Cancer as your rising sign, then this would be indicated by 'As', meaning 'ascendant', in the Cancer box on the chart and, depending on the source, a diagonal line may be added to that box to indicate the ascendant. This is also known as your *Lagna or* 'rising sign'. You may use this template to fill in your planetary positions to help you become familiar with your horoscope.

South Indian Birth Chart Layout

PISCES	ARIES	TAURUS	GEMINI
AQUARIUS			CANCER
CAPRICORN			LEO
SAGITTARIUS	SCORPIO	LIBRA	VIRGO

Fig. 1 South Indian Style Chart with Names of Signs in English.

Nature of the Signs

The Signs of the Zodiac

Sign	Quality	Dominant Element	Humour	Ruling Planet	Orientation	Body Part
Aries	Active	Fire	Fire	Mars (Inert)	Masculine	Head, brain, nerves
Taurus	Inert	Earth	Water	Venus (Active)	Feminine	Face, nose, eyes, mouth (teeth, tongue, oral cavity), throat
Gemini	Harmon-ious	Air	Air	Mercury (Active)	Masculine	Neck, shoulders, clavicles, arms, hands,
Cancer	Active	Water	Water/ Air	Moon (Harmoni ous)	Feminine	Heart, breast, chest, lungs
Leo	Inert	Fire	Fire	Sun (Harmon-ious)	Masculine	Solar plexus, heart, stomach, liver, gallbladder, spleen, duodenum, small intestines
Virgo	Harmon-ious	Earth	Air/ Water	Mercury (Active)	Feminine	Lower abdomen, large intestines
Libra	Active	Air	Air/ Water	Venus (Active)	Masculine	Pelvic region, urinary tract, kidneys, uterus, ovaries, bladder
Scorpio	Inert	Water	Water/ Fire	Mars & Ketu (Inert)	Feminine	Genitals, anus
Sagittarius	Harmon-ious	Fire	Fire/ Water	Jupiter (Harmon-ious)	Masculine	Hips, thighs, sciatic nerve
Capricorn	Active	Earth	Air/ Water	Saturn (Inert)	Feminine	Knees
Aquarius	Inert	Air	Air	Saturn & Rahu (Inert)	Masculine	Calves, shins, ankles
Pisces	Harmon-ious	Water	Water	Jupiter (Harmon-ious)	Feminine	Feet

Each sign is movable, fixed or dual in nature. In other words, each sign is active, inert or harmonious. This shows the nature of a sign, which is also modified according to the planet that rules it and by any planets you may have placed therein. The nature of each planet will show the intrinsic nature of the sign it rules while the actual outer nature of that sign is seen as whether it is active, inert or harmonious. Using the sign Taurus as an example, we can see that its outer nature is inert as it is a fixed sign. However, its ruler is the active planet Venus, which shows a more internal nature of the sign. How this plays out in life is that a Taurus influence will show a steadiness in achieving goals. The end result is harmonious, where peace and contentment are possible for those with this sign strongly influencing.

In the table of the Signs of the Zodiac provided, you will see that each sign is active, inert or harmonious, and each ruling planet is also active, inert or harmonious. When there is inertia upon inertia, as with the signs Scorpio and Aquarius, then the only possibility is inertia. When there is harmony upon harmony, then the result is also harmony, as seen in the signs Sagittarius and Pisces. When a sign is harmonious and its ruler is active, as in the case of Mercury's signs, Gemini and Virgo, then the ideals of the sign are not lived up to by the agitated Mercury and the end result is a breakdown into inertia. Harmony can only be arrived at with harmony, or when there are fewer objectives and lots of energy to achieve these objectives. Such is the case with the signs Aries, Taurus and Capricorn. When the rising sign is known, this alone can say a lot about your nature.

The table of signs provides only general indications as each sign's ruling planet would need to be looked at to take a more in-depth view.

Sign Interaction

Nothing is viewed in isolation so we need to see how the signs interact with one another. One way to do this is to look at the sign influences or aspects. These are a constant influence in your life, and any planets placed in a sign having an aspect on another will have an influence on that area of your life for the duration of your life. We will look at this interaction in relation to your first house only and the planets that have an influence on your nature. This shows which of the three qualities you express more in general terms. There are also planetary aspects that show more of an internal picture and are activated in periods of that planet. These are temporary influences that are triggered by these planetary periods, which show current imbalances. For now, we will look only at sign aspects and their effect on your nature from birth, which represents a constant influence throughout your life based on your constitution.

Sign Aspects

PISCES Dual Water-dominant	ARIES Movable Fire-dominant	TAURUS Fixed Earth-dominant	GEMINI Dual Air-dominant
AQUARIUS Fixed Air-dominant			CANCER Movable Water-dominant
CAPRICORN Movable Earth-dominant			LEO Fixed Fire-dominant
SAGITTARIUS Dual Fire-dominant	SCORPIO Fixed Water-dominant	LIBRA Movable Air-dominant	VIRGO Dual Earth-dominant

Fig 2. South Indian Style Chart with Zodiac Signs and their Nature

The movable signs aspect, or influence, the fixed signs, except the one beside it, and vice versa. The dual signs influence each other.

Using the south Indian chart layout in Fig. 2, you can see how the sign aspects look in a chart. The four corners are the dual signs of Gemini, Virgo, Sagittarius and Pisces.

The dual signs have a constant influence on each other, so that anyone with their rising sign in any of these will have the other three influence their sign. If there are planets placed in any of the other dual signs, then these will have an impact on their constitution. Another way to see a person's nature is to look at the 4th, 7th and 10th houses, along with the 1st house or rising sign, to see an influence from these. These four pillars of the chart are very influential, not merely in terms of constitutional analysis. The first house represents the self, the 4th represents the home, the 7th represents relationships and the 10th represents career. These are the four main pillars of life, upon which everything else is built. This influence is easy to see using the four dual signs in the chart in Fig. 2 because the four corner signs are influenced by the other elements placed in the 4th, 7th and 10th houses from that sign. So a person with the air sign Gemini as their rising sign will also have the other elements of earth, fire and water influence the sign from the 4th, 7th and 10th houses of Virgo, Sagittarius and Pisces.

It becomes somewhat more complicated if we take the movable and fixed signs in order to apply the same principles. Let us take Aries as an example of a movable sign. The fixed signs will influence it, i.e., the signs Leo, Scorpio and Aquarius, though not the fixed sign Taurus, as it is placed beside it. If we also take into account the 4th, 7th and 10th houses from the sign Aries, we also see the signs Cancer, Libra and Capricorn having an influence on the sign. Let us only take these angular houses (4, 7, and 10) into account if there are planets placed in these signs. The 10th house angle has the strongest influence, followed by the 7th and then the 4th. If there are no planets contained in any of these houses, then we can take only the fixed sign influence and look at the planets placed therein. If there were no planets involved in the picture, either in the fixed signs or the movable signs, we could see nature as a perfect balance of the elements, and this balance would be expressed in nature. However, it is the planets which bring imbalances into our lives so that we may live out the results of our previous thoughts, words and actions through these imbalances.

If we take the sign Taurus as the rising sign, then the movable signs of Cancer, Libra and Capricorn will influence this sign throughout life. The signs of Leo, Scorpio and Aquarius will impact if there are planets placed therein. So using this example, if the sign Leo had Saturn placed therein, and the sign Aquarius housed the planet Jupiter, we can see that the nature of this individual born with Taurus rising would reflect the influence of both Saturn and Jupiter. In other words, this individual will have the influence of air and water in their constitutional makeup. If there are no fiery planets influencing the first house, or the ruler of the first house, (in this case, Venus), then there will not be a strong fire type.

Though these general rules apply, as with everything, each individual must be looked at more specifically. Nothing in life is ever viewed as completely independent so it is no different with the study of the horoscope. Everything has an impact on everything else. Keep this in mind when beginning to study your own nature as seen in your own horoscope. No book can give you the exact, in-depth analysis required for such a study. We are all complex beings, and though generalities can always be applied – even though you know it does not describe the whole picture – you can still use the knowledge gained to further understand your place within nature.

Summary of Aspects

In short, the movable signs look at the fixed signs, thus influencing them, while the fixed signs look at the movable signs, except for the adjacent signs. The dual signs, which have the balance between both movable and fixed qualities, influence each other. The planets in the 1st, 4th, 7th and 10th houses will influence if there are any planets placed therein, especially the 1st, followed by the 10th, 7th and 4th houses. It makes sense if you apply this to a typical scenario in life we all come in contact with. Let us take an example of a chart that has a fixed sign rising (Taurus, Leo, Scorpio or Aquarius). These signs will have a movable 9th house (count 9 signs from any fixed sign and you will arrive at a movable sign). The 9th house represents the father and one's teachers. In this way, we see the father and/or teachers getting the individual to move, and allowing them to aspire for greater things, while the individual themselves, as a fixed sign, can be seen as holding the father and/or teachers back in some way. This is, of course, a very simplified way to see how signs interact and would need further scrutiny in a horoscope.

Another example using an Ayurvedic approach could be seen in someone who is hyperactive by nature and needing some herbs or foods that slow them down. If we are out of balance, then we seek things that bring us further out of balance. To find balance once again, we must seek things that offer an opposing quality to bring us into harmony. So again, we see the need to achieve a balanced state of being. This is no different when considering an exercise that is suitable to an individual's needs. We need to acknowledge and work constantly within activity and inactivity, which naturally balance each other but they are, in and of themselves, that which cause imbalances. We are striving to maintain a more balanced life, which really means finding a balance between inactivity and activity and the resulting better health.

From the previous chart of zodiac signs and their nature (Fig. 2), we can see that nature has perfect balance without the inclusion of the planetary influences. When we add these planets, we can see how a person's nature is an expression of imbalance as a soul's need to live out the results of its previous thoughts, words and actions through the influence of the planets. It is the planets that hold these imprints on the soul and make sure we live out these by bringing imbalances into our nature as well as becoming imbalanced within the scope of our given nature.

Sample Chart Analysis

PISCES 5	ARIES 6 Mars RX	TAURUS 7	GEMINI 8 Ketu (The South Node) Saturn RX
AQUARIUS 4	**Natal Chart** The Author Born Monday, 22 October 1973 12.53pm GMT Leeds, UK		CANCER 9
CAPRICORN 3 Jupiter	RX = Retrograde		LEO 10 Moon
SAGITTARIUS 2 Rahu (The North Node)	SCORPIO 1 Ascendant Venus	LIBRA 12 Sun Mercury	VIRGO 11

Fig. 3 Author's Birth Chart

In Fig. 3, the example given is of the author's birth chart using the south Indian-style chart. In this chart layout, the signs do not move and are as per the previous template given, with Pisces in the top left-hand corner and Aries to its right. Counting 8 signs from Aries (the natural first house), we can see the rising sign is Scorpio with 'Ascendant' placed in the sign. This becomes the first house for this horoscope.

Analysis of Qualities

From the Signs of the Zodiac table, you can see that Scorpio is inert in nature. This is because Scorpio is a fixed sign (as shown in the Sign Aspects chart) and ruled by Mars and Ketu – both destructive (inert) planets. Venus is in the rising sign and is active in nature. However, it is placed in an inert sign and is influenced by Mars' aspect from the sign Aries. In addition, this birth chart is influenced by a debilitated Jupiter as it is placed in its sign of debilitation, Capricorn. Debilitated planets are more inert in nature and exalted planets are more harmonious in nature, so here Jupiter becomes more inert. Taking the planetary ruler into account, we see that Ketu (the south node) is placed with a planet (Saturn) in Gemini, and Mars is on its own in the sign Aries. Any time a decision has to be made as to which ruler to use, the planet taken into account is the one placed with more planets. This will occur only in the case of the rising signs Scorpio and Aquarius, which both have two rulers (see Signs of the Zodiac table). In this case, Ketu is taken as the first house ruler in this initial analysis of constitution. Ketu is placed in the sign Gemini and is being influenced by the inert planet Saturn, by its placement alongside it. The overall result is of inertia with some activity.

You may wonder how it is that a more inert individual would end up writing a book about exercise according to astrological principles! Firstly, when analysing the nature, we cannot simply view the natal chart alone, even though this is telling. We must also view the 9th divisional chart to see the intrinsic nature on a deeper level. It is true that this author is at times more inert, but this has led to periods of activity that have led to lifestyles incorporating physical exercises such as dance from an early age, leading to yogic practices later in life. Yoga suits as an exercise as it offers an experience of inactivity within physical activity as well as balancing for the dominant air and fire humours, which we will look at subsequently. Note also the inclusion of Venus in the rising sign, which gives an overall feeling of comfort and, at times, an indulgent nature. Even the spirit of this book has been to access the body's innate intelligence, which is an inert substance in and of itself.

We must also remember that the qualities are impulses we can work with and change as well as there being a natural cycle of these within our lifetime. Along with awareness and right lifestyle choices, we can, with effort, change the quality of our experience. However, we cannot alter our nature in terms of the biological humours. The balance you were born with stays with you for life, whether you remain in balance with this or not.

Analysis of the Humours

Scorpio is a water-dominant sign and is ruled by Mars, which represents the fire element. This combines the elements of water and fire in an inert sign. However, we could not simply stop there with the analysis, even though on one level this in itself is very telling of the nature of the author. We must see the planets influencing the sign and the ruler of the sign, which in this case has two – namely Mars and Ketu. They are both 'fiery' in nature. We have already seen that Ketu is taken into account more prominently for constitutional analysis. It is placed with the 'airy' planet Saturn, in an air-dominant sign Gemini. This gives a strong air indication along with fire.

The waning Moon (air) in the 10th house will also influence the nature, along with Venus (air and water) strongly influencing in the 1st house. These bring more of an air influence, with a weaker water influence due to influences upon Venus. A strongly placed Mars in 'trinal' strength (see Trinal Strength table) influencing Scorpio, and Venus placed therein, indicates more fire. Jupiter is also influencing Scorpio, which would ordinarily show more of a water-dominant nature. However, Jupiter is debilitated in the sign Capricorn and so the influence of water is not as strong as it would be if it were in another sign.

Looking at just the static analysis, we can see that there is more of an air and fire influence on the nature of the author. This is the constitution according to this chart analysis and this has been confirmed by Ayurvedic doctors many times. The water nature that is an expression of the water-dominant sign Scorpio is not being expressed as strongly as another individual with this rising sign, and without these planetary influences.

Weekday Ruling Planet

One way to quickly see the constitution is to study the planet that rules the day on which you were born. In the chart given, the weekday at birth was Monday, which is the Moon's day (the weekday is taken from sunrise to sunrise). The position and relevant biological humour can then be studied by the strength and position of that planet. If the planet in question is strong, then it bodes well for the physical strength of the native. In the example chart, the Moon as the ruler of the day of week is not without some hindrances. It is placed in a friendly and prominent 10th house, in the sign Leo, which is ruled by the Sun. The Moon is weaker because it is waning, i.e., moving towards the Sun (the Moon wanes when it moves from the 7th to 1st house position from the Sun), indicating an air humour as already seen in the previous analysis. The fire humour comes from its position in Leo, which is a fire-dominant sign. The ruler of Leo is the debilitated Sun in Libra, which creates an underlying weakness in the constitution despite any strength of the Moon in the chart. This is not only due to the Sun's representation of overall vitality, but because in this instance it rules the sign that the Moon (the day ruler) is placed in.

Taking the planet that rules the day of the week on which you were born, you will be able to ascertain the strength or weakness of this planet according to the tables given. Take note of the planet that rules the sign in which your ruling weekday ruler sits as this will give you more of an understanding of an underlying strength or weakness.

The 9th Divisional Chart

The 9th divisional chart (Fig. 4) is known as the *Navamsha,* or D-9, and is studied alongside the main *Rasi* or 'birth chart', which we have hitherto looked at for constitutional analysis. The 9th division simply divides the signs of the main birth chart further into nine sections per sign, giving us another chart to study. This chart also gives clues as to the nature of an individual by taking a deeper look at the strengths and weaknesses of the planets as well as looking at the chart as a whole alongside the main birth chart.

In a study of the author's nature, we will only concern ourselves with the rising sign in this 9th harmonic chart, which in this case is the sign Pisces. Jupiter is placed in strength in its own sign Pisces, which would indicate a more harmonious constitution. However, because of Jupiter's debilitation in the main birth chart, it is not able to express its harmonious nature physically. In other words, though there may be a more harmonious temperament, because of Jupiter's debility in the main chart, there is a lack of a physically harmonious constitution, which leads to weakness. The main chart is concerned with the physical body primarily as well as the general circumstances in life. The divisional charts each look at specific areas of life in more detail. There are sixteen of these divisional charts that are examined in an individual's horoscope. The 9th division is the most important to look at in any chart interpretation and is always given alongside the main birth chart for any analysis. One cannot be studied without the other. You will not arrive at a well-rounded picture without the 9th divisional chart.

PISGES 1 Ascendant Jupiter	ARIES 2	TAURUS 3	GEMINI 4 Mercury Mars Rx The North Node
AQUARIUS 12	**Ninth Divisional Chart** The Author Born 22 October 1973 12.53pm GMT Leeds, UK		CANCER 5
CAPRICORN 11 Saturn Rx Venus	Rx = Retrograde		LEO 6
SAGITTARIUS 10 The South Node	SCORPIO 9 Sun	LIBRA 8 Moon	VIRGO 7

Fig. 4 - 9th Divisional Chart

As you can see, the analysis of a particular individual's nature from the birth chart is a complex study. The example given is itself a very simplified view and does not include many other indications and areas of study required. The reason for giving such an example is not to confuse the reader, but to show how there is a complex interpretation that needs further investigation. The aim of this book is to begin that investigation for yourself by gradually building up a picture of your unique nature. Though you may be able to say you are someone with the sign Gemini rising, there is a more intricate portrait of that sign for you than of someone else with the same rising sign. At the same time, you can acknowledge your nature according to whatever sign is rising in your horoscope.

Your Horoscope

PISCES	ARIES	TAURUS	GEMINI
AQUARIUS	**Birth Chart**		CANCER
CAPRICORN			LEO
SAGITTARIUS	SCORPIO	LIBRA	VIRGO

Fig. 5 – Your Birth Chart

Your 9th Divisional Chart

PISCES	ARIES	TAURUS	GEMINI
AQUARIUS	**9th Divisional Chart**		CANCER
CAPRICORN			LEO
SAGITTARIUS	SCORPIO	LIBRA	VIRGO

Fig. 6 – The 9th Divisional Chart

Having obtained the planetary positions from your horoscope, first of all take note of the rising sign and fill this in using the template birth chart provided in Fig. 5, or by drawing this template for yourself. You may indicate your rising sign by using a diagonal line through the box or by placing the number **1** inside. Then take note of any planets that may be placed in that sign and write them in. Fill in the rest of the positions of the planets. Take note of the planet that rules your 1st house as seen in the Signs of the Zodiac table given earlier. Now you have two important pieces of information – your rising sign and its nature, and your ruling planet and its nature. Look to see where that planet is placed in your chart by sign and house placement by filling in the rest of the planetary positions through all of the houses.

Now take a look at the aspects to your rising sign and to your ruling planet. Remember the rule that the fixed signs aspect the movable signs and vice versa, except the sign adjacent. The dual signs aspect one another. As you build up a picture of your nature in the chart, start noting how many times air, fire and water occur in your analysis, and which is more prominent, writing down each time you notice an influence of each. You should begin to see a correlation between what you are finding here with the Ayurvedic questionnaire you filled out with your whole life in mind.

You can then do the same for the 9th divisional chart. This will give you a more in-depth look at your nature as everything in this chart will deepen your awareness alongside the main birth chart. The 9th divisional chart is a more detailed analysis of the strengths and weaknesses of each of the planets and is taken into account along with the main birth chart as well as a separate chart. For now, you may simply work with only the main chart and use the 9th divisional chart's rising sign.

NB. You will need to be working with an exact time of birth in order for the 9th divisional chart to be accurate as the rising sign in this chart changes approximately every 15 minutes.

Masculine and Feminine Signs and Planets

Count how many planets you have in fire-, earth-, air- and water-dominant signs. Air- and fire-dominant signs are masculine in nature, and earth- and water-dominant signs are feminine in nature. Though you may have a feminine sign as your rising sign, along with a more feminine planet placed therein, you may also have more planets in masculine signs overall, or vice versa. This may mean you are more masculine or feminine in nature, but have a different orientation overall, especially when taking your Moon and Sun signs into account and the core of your being.

Each of the five planets – Mercury, Venus, Mars, Jupiter and Saturn – has both a masculine and feminine sign through which they find expression. However, in and of themselves, the planets are either more masculine or feminine. The feminine planets are Venus, the Moon and Rahu. The masculine planets are the Sun, Jupiter, Mars and Ketu. Saturn and Mercury are seen as neutral, so you do not have to include them in this type of analysis for now. Mercury becomes more influenced by the sign it is placed in and the planets it is placed alongside.

Take note of how many times you notice feminine signs housing feminine planets and masculine signs housing masculine planets. Do this with regards to your first house initially, as this will indicate whether your nature is either more assertive (masculine) or receptive (feminine). If a masculine sign also has a masculine planet placed therein, then this shows even more of an assertive expression in such a case. If this is so in the case of your rising sign, then your nature is more masculine-oriented. The same is true if a feminine sign has a feminine planet placed therein.

A Breathing Exercise

The masculine and feminine influence is one that changes throughout our life as well as being a constant influence, depending on your horoscope. This variance is due to planetary periods and transits, and their influence on our current nature. Overall, however, there is a predominance of either a masculine or feminine nature. Along with your chart analysis, you may also try a breathing exercise that can help you ascertain the predominance in any given moment.

Steady the mind on the breath for a few cycles of breathing. Spend longer at this if your mind is more disturbed. If your mind is too disturbed, you may put off this exercise for a more appropriate time. Notice if you are more comfortable with the space at the end of the inhales or at the end of the exhales. If you are more comfortable with the fullness at the end of the inhales, then you are more identified with life and the feminine expression of your being. If this is an ongoing experience, then you are more identified with the water- and earth-dominant signs and the more feminine planets. If you are more comfortable at the end of the exhales, there can be a complete sense of letting go and relaxation. At that moment, you are more identified with the masculine expression of your being. If this is more of an ongoing experience, then you are more influenced with the fire- and air-dominant signs as well as the masculine-oriented planets.

CHAPTER 5 - HEAVENLY BODIES

The planet that rules your first house is paramount in relation to your overall health and well-being (see the Signs of the Zodiac table in the previous chapter). Knowing your ruling planet deepens your awareness of your nature. The signs themselves are the planet's way of expressing themselves through us. The houses show the areas in our life in which they find their expression. Knowing the nature of the planet that rules your rising sign will add greatly to your awareness of your own nature. Because you embody that planet in a physical sense, as well as your characteristics, you can become more conscious of how you find expression of this planet by studying it in your horoscope.

We will now look at each of the planets and how to acknowledge each of them in your life and exercise routines. Although you may not have any planets placed in your first house, you will benefit from reading about all of the planets. You still have a mind (Moon) and an identity (Sun) to balance in order to remain healthy. You need to express your physical energy (Mars) and learn lessons which you can apply practically (Mercury) to any exercise you choose. You need to develop a more intuitive awareness of safe movement (Jupiter), and love your body and its ability to naturally find balance (Venus). You must also meet with very necessary restrictions as you learn to let go of any attachments to an end result when you work out (Saturn). You are constantly evolving in your routines (Rahu) while you grow from territory you have already conquered (Ketu) – making peace with where you have come from.

All of the planets represent energies that are alive in you, expressing their nature through you. They do this in different ways for each of us and by varying degrees, based on their influence in the chart. The Sun and Moon, all the planets and the nodes of the Moon (Rahu and Ketu) represent certain things for all of us and specific things for each of us. Following is a description of those certain things they represent for all of us. To know what each planet represents for you specifically, you must study your horoscope to see the signs, and therefore the areas (house positions), they represent for you. Refer back to the table of planets and signs given and consult with your own horoscope.

The Planets and the Tissues of the Body

In *Brihat Parasara Hora Shastra*, the most comprehensive text on Vedic astrology, by the Indian sage Parasara, it states that 'bones, blood, marrow, skin, fat, semen and muscles are the primary ingredients' and that 'the lords of these are respectively the Sun and the other planets'. Therefore, bones are ruled by the Sun, blood by the Moon, marrow by Mars, skin and plasma by Mercury, fat by Jupiter, reproductive fluid by Venus and muscle by Saturn. This gives great insight into the workings of the body when viewing the position and strength of each planet in the horoscope in order to ascertain the strength or weakness of a particular tissue in the body. Bodily organs also correspond to each of the planets and, of course, groups of organs make up systems in the body. This corresponds to the intricate interplay between systems in the body and the planets in the horoscope.

The Sun represents the ruling force in the horoscope which represents the skeleton of the body – that which holds us up – just as our star keeps the planets spinning in space. The bones are nourished by blood, represented by the Moon, which is the nurturing force in the horoscope. The muscles (Saturn) do the work of moving the bones. Mars represents the nerves, which give the order to the muscles to move, while Mercury relays this message throughout the body. The fat and fluids are represented by the benevolent planets – Jupiter, the Moon, Venus and Mercury, which protect the body and maintain homeostasis.

The Sun

The Sun is the centre of our solar system and in the horoscope it represents the centre of our being. It is representative of spirit – the one spirit we all share. Every time we engage in a spiritual practice, or we experience a physical exercise as a spiritual experience, we are engaging with that Higher Self. We strengthen our connection to our true source of power and we build confidence and self-esteem as a result. All the planets revolve around the Sun as it holds everything in place, just as our sense of self and self-esteem hold everything in place for us. The Sun represents the bone tissue – the Sun's gravitational pull of the planets reflecting our own skeleton's ability to hold our bodies upright.

The Sun, being the centre of the solar system, rules all things in positions of importance like governments and people in authority. Individuals with a strong Sun in their horoscope have a strong sense of self and identity. These individuals are usually in positions of power. It is when this is afflicted in some way that we see ego problems. Ego problems can occur with a weak Sun, just as a weak individual who plays the martyr in order to develop a stronger sense of self. A healthy, balanced Sun represents a healthy, balanced ego. A healthy ego takes its strength from a higher sense of Self.

The paths of yoga and Ayurveda are that of toning the ego and can sometimes result in difficulty gaining access to a Higher Self. However, these paths offer a way through the ego and beyond, like a bridge to something greater than us. Those on the path of hatha yoga should be aware of the pitfalls involved. Achieving a great feat in a yoga posture massages not only the internal organs! This is the danger that all yogis should be aware of in their practice. When we achieve any sense of connection to this power, and we go with the flow of life as we were meant to, our ego can sometimes lay claim to having accomplished it. Yet, we have merely let things happen as they are meant to. We align ourselves with our soul's purpose. This empowering sense of self can so easily be hijacked by the ego. Having a strong Sun with malefic influences can create these kinds of challenges. Likewise, someone with a weak Sun will compensate for this, and though they may appear weak, the ego is strengthened by playing the martyr.

When the Sun is weakly placed in the horoscope, there can be humility, but there can also be a lack of self-esteem and confidence. There is a fine line between humility and low self-esteem, and those with a weak Sun will be very familiar with walking that line. Individuals with a debilitated Sun may have a great ability to be humbled in life, whereas those with an exalted Sun may never be able to get on to their knees when a certain life experience is asking this of them.

Individuals with a weak Sun energy can work at strengthening this quality if they are to become comfortable with their power and their light in the world. You may have the Sun in debility, but it is not the full picture and needs more scrutiny from a full horoscope analysis. However, if your Sun is weak, you will have to address the issue of a lack of confidence and self-esteem to some degree. You may back the underdog as you will see in those less fortunate or able a quality in yourself that you can easily relate to. An individual with a weak solar energy will often have difficulty with authoritative figures, i.e., people with a strongly placed Sun, but there is also an attraction to them. A planet in debility will always be opposite to its exaltation position in the chart. This shows how we can look to those for that which we lack ourselves. For those with a weak Sun, it is advisable to literally get some sun. It is beneficial for them to come to terms with and respect authority and their own connection to a Higher Self, especially when relating to others. People with a strong Sun may not need to strengthen this energy, but rather purify it, remaining humble under the gaze of such a powerful luminary.

The Sun and the Body

The Sun has the qualities of promoting a connection to a Higher Self, is luminous, upward moving and cosmically intelligent. However, it is also seen as malefic because of its burning effect. Physically getting a little Sun is beneficial, but too much and you will burn. The Sun is seen in Ayurveda as balanced fire if it is well placed in the horoscope. It causes heat in the body that is health promoting, such as a healthy digestive fire. With a strong Sun, there is robust health, whereas a weak Sun will show poor health overall. According to Parasara: 'The Sun has honey coloured eyes, square body, he is of clean habits, is bilious, intelligent, manly and has limited hair on his head.' The Sun represents the bones, the heart, stomach and the right eye. Afflictions to the Sun can cause any number of diseases owing to its general signification of health and vitality, but more specific diseases caused are heart, eye, bone disease and conditions relating to the spine.

The Sun and the Spine

The Sun shows our ability to stand (or sit) tall. Someone with an afflicted Sun in the horoscope will not only have issues around confidence, but may also feel the effects of this physically in the spine. When there is a lack of self-esteem and confidence, the shoulders tend to slump forward and the chest drops as if to hide from the world. This posture will have an effect on the spine. If someone has a severe affliction to the Sun and other indications involving the 8th house of their horoscope, that individual may have been born with a lack of integrity in the spine. Some spinal conditions can be rectified with awareness and postural work as well as the Sun salutations used in hatha yoga. Sun salutations flex and strengthen the spine, offering individuals their own corrective postural work. Having a daily practice of greeting the Sun and your Higher Self on the yoga mat, in meditation or in whatever form of exercise or activity you are engaged in, is of the utmost importance to someone with a weak solar energy. Those with a weak solar energy often feel more confident when they have a physical exercise routine that gives them a stronger sense of self.

With a weakly placed Sun, there can be a need to compensate for a feeling of lack. This may result in puffing out the chest in order to stand taller, exaggerating oneself in order to seem more important. In such a case, the spine still suffers due to the strain. It can be seen that a middle ground needs to be explored through a lengthening of the spine before lifting the chest and standing or sitting tall. You will fool no one when pretending to be something you are not. Eventually through whatever exercise you choose, you may arrive at a place of quiet confidence where there is no need for showing off with grand gestures – only a strong yet humble sense of self. This will then be expressed in a healthy, flexible spine.

Exercise for the Sun

Any exercise that is rhythmic in nature is beneficial for our health. Exercises like dance, running or sports that have a sense of rhythm are all good, though rhythm can be cultivated in any form of exercise. Hatha yoga's Sun salutations, in particular, are a very beneficial exercise for the spine. They comprise a 12-pose series performed together with the breath as a flowing movement and were traditionally practiced 12 times – once for each sign of the zodiac. In addition, they were traditionally practised while facing east each morning as the Sun rose. They dispel the three humours from the spine and stimulate circulation. These movements improve digestion, reduce weight, and promote youth and vitality. As the Sun is representative of our confidence and vitality, working with this awareness and intention can add to the effectiveness of your Sun salutations each morning. I would strongly encourage you to seek out a teacher to learn how to safely perform this invaluable set of exercises. All three of the biological humours benefit from this series of postures, though the way in which you approach the practice will depend on your body type as always (refer to the guidelines given for each humour).

The air types' anxious energy can be spent before allowing them to slow down and ground themselves in their movement. The fire types' outward drive can be facilitated before settling down into their bodies and allowing themselves to open gently in whatever routine they choose. The water types' energy needs this form of exercise to dispel lethargy and to get stagnant energy flowing once more.

Leo - Embodying the Sun

The house position of your Sun shows where in life you will need to find your unique ability to shine. The sign Leo, being an embodiment of the Sun, also becomes an area where you will find this need to express this light and power. You will have a need to be admired in this area of your life. Those with the sign Leo rising in their horoscope will no doubt have a need to shine, sometimes needing to be at the centre of attention, and have a powerful sense of self if there are no other indications suggesting otherwise.

Calculating your Sun Sign

Look at the house position of the Sun in your chart. It shows where you need to express your sense of true power and self-esteem. If there is a hindrance to this, then you will feel like your light is not being allowed to shine. If the Sun is placed in an active sign, there is more of an outward expression of the solar impulse. If it is placed in an inert sign, then this is applied more stubbornly than if it is placed in a harmonious sign, where it can be more adaptable. Look to see which element is dominant in your Sun sign as the three qualities of activity, harmony and inertia have their expression in all the elements. Look to see if it is placed in a masculine or feminine sign, as this will show either a more assertive or passive quality. If, for example, the Sun were placed in Aries, which is a fire-dominant, masculine sign, there is much more of a dynamic quality to the Sun than that of a Sun placed in the sign Cancer, which is a water-dominant, feminine sign. The Sun is also exalted in Aries, which means it is able to express its strength if there are no other obstructions. It is seen as debilitated in the sign opposite in Libra, where one feels humbled.

Sun in Aries	April 14 to May 13
Sun in Taurus	May 14 to June 13
Sun in Gemini	June 14 to July 15
Sun in Cancer	July 16 to August 15
Sun in Leo	August 16 to September 15
Sun in Virgo	September 16 to October 16
Sun in Libra	October 17 to November 15
Sun in Scorpio	November 16 to December 14
Sun in Sagittarius	December 15 to January 13
Sun in Capricorn	January 14 to February 12
Sun in Aquarius	February 13 to March 13
Sun in Pisces	March 14 to April 13

Monthly Solar Ingress

The date of the month the Sun moves signs in the sidereal zodiac, as used in Vedic astrology, differs from that of the view of the tropical zodiac, which is used by most modern Western astrologers. These dates may also change by a day, depending on your location. If your birthday is on the dates the Sun changes sign, it is best to check with a Vedic astrologer or astrology resource in order to ascertain your correct Sun sign.

The Moon

Most of us are aware of the Moon, if only by looking up at the night sky during a full Moon night. Awareness of the Moon's influence on our emotional body is also prevalent. We may all have been witness to a certain 'lunacy' in some around the time of the full Moon or we may be aware of the Moon's role in a woman's monthly cycle. The Moon's cycles are literally at the heart of our lives. In Vedic astrology, many times the Moon is studied before anything else because it shows how we feel about anything – our likes and dislikes. The Moon represents our mind and emotions as well as our senses and sense of well-being. It represents our mother and home environment – the home we feel within ourselves. In other words, it represents our sense of peace and security.

The Moon represents our overall mind but, more specifically, our subconscious mind. It represents our instinctual nature, as opposed to Mercury, which represents the rational thinking mind. A well-placed Moon with benevolent influences will show an emotionally strong individual and is preferable for an individual's mental and emotional health. Such a placement will positively affect the physical health also. A weakly placed Moon with malevolent influences will show challenges to our sense of well-being, a poor mental and emotional health, and lead to poor physical health. The light of the Sun is reflected in the Moon, which has no light of its own. This represents the universal self – reflected in the individuated self. A strong Sun energy can go a long way to alleviate mental and emotional challenges. This factor reflects the ability for exercise, if observed routinely, to alleviate many of our mental and emotional challenges.

In Vedic astrology, there are 27 lunar signs, or constellations, that are studied for analysis of an individual's psychological makeup. They have their roots in a more ancient lunar zodiac as it was the Moon along with the Sun that ancient peoples first looked to for calculating time. While in Western astrology, the use of the Sun sign calculation is widespread and applied so generally so as to invalidate the use of astrology altogether, in the Eastern sidereal zodiac, an individual's Moon sign is used to see a person's psychological state as well as other general and physical traits. Though a study of these influences is not under the scope of this book, it is also possible to see the impact of the lunar signs on constitution.

The Moon is new when it reaches the same degree as the Sun in the zodiac and is full when it is opposite to the Sun. It is said to be more malevolent when it is waning (moving towards the Sun) and more benevolent when it is waxing (moving away from the Sun). Activities should always be performed with respect to the position and cycles of the Moon along with the Sun. Just as the Sun and Moon give us life, as our Father and Mother, our luminaries continually do so by their influence upon life on Earth. The Sun's distance from Earth is 108 times its diameter just as the Moon's distance from Earth is 108 times its diameter. The Moon's influence is needed for life to exist on Earth.

Certain activities are more desirable when the Moon is in certain constellations; likewise, during certain transits of the Moon, certain activities should not be performed. In general, auspicious activities should begin during the waxing phase of the Moon and a more introspective approach is cultivated during the waning phase. Very simply, you may think of something you would like to grow during the fortnight of the waxing Moon and something to let go of in the waning phase. In Horary astrology, where an optimal time is chosen to perform a certain activity, it is the Moon and its signs that hold great importance, although they are not the only prerequisite.

Meditation strengthens the mind and calms the emotions, helping us to deal with certain emotions that seem insurmountable at times. The type of meditation one performs will show what is being increased in the mind. A silent meditation increases the element of space in the mind, leading to a feeling of spaciousness. Meditations that are more focused and concentrated on an object will increase the fire in the mind, leading to clarity. Meditations on the heart are the easiest way to access the Moon and the Self, such as Loving Kindness Meditation, leading to feelings of peace and contentment.

The Moon and the Body

The Moon rules the blood tissue, lymph, breasts, uterus, ovaries, mucous membranes and the left eye. It rules over the fluids in the body, and any difficulties with these are indicated by a disturbance to the Moon. Mental and emotional problems are the result of an afflicted Moon. In *Brihat Parasara Hora Shastra,* the sage Parasara describes the Moon as 'very windy and phlegmatic. She has a round body and is learned. She has auspicious looks and sweet speech, is fickle-minded and very lustful.' It is more 'airy' when waning and more 'watery' when it is waxing. Our bodies are more than 70 per cent water, depending on our age, and the Moon's influence on the water content in our bodies is seen by its position at birth as well as being an ongoing phenomenon.

Exercise for the Moon

Exercise with the Moon in mind could flow more, allowing anything that the body wishes to feel in the moment to be felt fully. We seek to busy the mind with physical activity and, in doing so; we slowly quieten it enough so that we can access our true nature, beyond any emotional upset or thought processes. Whatever form of exercise you engage in would ideally involve your absolute presence for this to occur. Otherwise, you may find your mind just as busy in a routine it can perform automatically. This is why we experience such a sense of calm when we first try out new exercises or routines that require our complete focus and why many engage in dangerous activities and extreme sports. Our minds have to be more focused on the exercise and not on our everyday worries and anxieties.

For most, the experience of the Moon, and therefore of their sense of self, is through thoughts and emotions. On a deeper level, when we connect with our true Self, there is a stillness that is impossible to put into words. We touch a place in our being that is beyond any thoughts or emotions, and this expresses our true nature better than any words could. Yet this Self is an individuated Self and only a reflection of our true source of power and true spirit. We get a sense of the oneness of our true spirit now and then, but this is beyond even approaching a satisfactory description. Once one attempts such a description, the experience of oneness itself has disappeared.

Simply observing the breath has a quietening effect on the mind as we are taken into the present moment and feeling whatever emotions are moving through us. A meditative exercise routine allows these feelings to come up and be processed, without the need to react. Any exercise will allow your mind to settle into the body and instead of suppressing the emotion, you allow it to pass through, which is all that an emotion wishes to do. Exercising with this in mind allows you to work with the energy without suppression, but also without getting into a reactive state with what is going on inside you. Instead, you may observe your need to react and how this manifests in the body.

If the mind is too disturbed to concentrate on an exercise or activity, then just lying on props in order to gently expand the chest can be beneficial. In this way, you can still exercise the body in a passive way by opening it up and stretching it gently. You can then observe how you are feeling in the safety of your own space. The body can then become a sanctuary for you if you need it. The more you exercise or meditate, the more of your energy and intention go into it, making it a place you can delve safely into matters of the heart.

The Moon's Phases

When we become aware of the Moon's phases, we can plan exercise accordingly. *Ashtanga* Yoga practitioners are familiar with the new and full Moon days and do not practise on these two days of the month. This is because the extreme energy of the day is not conducive to such a high-energy practice. The new Moon day is reflective of low energy, which can be scattered, leading to a further drain of energy when exercising. The full Moon days are times when we literally feel full of ourselves and can lead to an exaggerated environment where we may push too hard and overdo it. It is best to hold back on such days and to exercise gently. Water types may find the full Moon days are more of a challenge due to the heaviness that is possible. Air types may feel more grounded, with a lot more energy and endurance. However, air types would still benefit from not overdoing things, no matter how loath they are to withhold energy. The new Moon days are times when we feel low in energy and, though water types may benefit from the lightness generated, it is generally a time to withhold and slow down.

Cancer - Embodying the Moon

If Cancer is your rising sign, then the Moon rules your first house and your sense of Self is greatly coloured by the Moon and its cycles. If this is not your rising sign, then the house position of Cancer as well as the position of the Moon in your horoscope will show areas of life in which you seek comfort. Those born with this sign rising must acknowledge the ebb and flow of their moods, addressing them in physical activities when the mood strikes. Otherwise, a 'Moon type' may plan routines though other considerations may become more pressing. Whether an individual can override how they are feeling in any given moment in order to exercise will depend on the position and strength of Mars in the horoscope.

The Moon is exalted in the sign of Taurus and debilitated in the opposite sign Scorpio. This cannot be taken as the only indication for the strength of the Moon (or for any planet), as there are a number of ways of calculating strength. However, if the Moon is debilitated, whether that has been cancelled out by something else or not, there will still be a need to meet this in life. The strength of the Moon is in finding comfort in family, food and security, our basic needs being met, as represented by its place of strength in Taurus. The weakness of the Moon is in feelings of insecurity, as we reach beyond comfort zones, researching the depths of our being – finding out what makes us tick. As intriguing a pursuit as this is, the mind does not feel safe and secure. The Moon in Scorpio shows an ability to think of the worst-case scenario and, in doing so, prepares the mind for such an event. The goal here is to find emotional strength ultimately, as represented by Scorpio's ruling planet Mars, the planet of courage and strength. However, the mind dwelling on such things will not feel safe and protected. If your Moon is placed in Scorpio, it is important to acknowledge your natural tendencies, but also balance them with what might be perceived as trivial pursuits or pleasures. For those with the Moon placed in Scorpio, these pursuits are anything but trivial, and are a very necessary part of a healthy, balanced mind.

Exaltation or debilitation should not be looked at as either 'good' or 'bad', as the mind would like to label it, but should be seen as a means to work with the impulse in your life. Having the Moon debilitated in Scorpio can show someone who has the ability to reach great depths and apply this to understanding the inner workings of the mind. Someone with the Moon exalted in Taurus may use the impulse of the Moon to create and look after a family or one's own community through food and other sustaining means. Remember that the Moon does not have a light of its own, but instead reflects the light of the Sun. Therefore, the Moon brings a need to connect with others and each other's light.

Calculating your Moon Sign

Look to see in which house your Moon is placed as this shows where you seek comfort. It shows where you experience the ever-changing phases of the Moon and subsequent changes in your life. The area of your life to which you apply this more changeable and emotional nature will be seen by the house position. If, for example, your Moon is placed in your first house, you may be changeable in nature and must acknowledge this when setting out an exercise strategy and timetable. Look to the house position of your Moon sign to see if you can relate this to your own need for comfort and security.

Mars

Mars represents our strength. It shows our ability to destroy that which is making us weak. This may mean performing exercises that require more strength and dexterity as well as a focusing of energy to accomplish a task or feat. Mars represents our physical prowess and ability to cut through something in order to remove obstacles. An athlete, a surgeon or a soldier (all 'Mars-type' individuals) cannot second guess what they are doing if they are to perform their tasks well. Mars' influence shows a lot of action without too much thought. It is because of this blind nature that it is seen as an inert planet, even though a strong Mars makes one very active, but without due consideration. A weak Mars can make one inactive and dull. A build-up of Mars energy, if not expressed or allowed a physical outlet, will manifest as toxic heat and can cause arguments, accidents and all sorts of problems. Even though you may achieve a lot of goals, physical activity is a better use of the Mars impulse than intellectual achievements alone.

Mars is a 'fiery' planet. It represents brute force and aggression, and a strong Mars in a horoscope will show the ability to stand up and fight. A strong Mars is necessary to have any get up and go. A weak Mars might make one timid and perhaps give a tendency to bottle up anger, which can then lead to all kinds of difficulties. This may also be expressed as if one had a very strong Mars, but this is a compensation for a weak Mars and is coming from a place of weakness. It is seen in many sporting greats that Mars is weakly placed in their horoscope, indicating the need to achieve even greater feats and successes due to this feeling of weakness. Many sporting greats have had to overcome tremendous challenges in order to excel in their chosen sport. If you were born with a weak limb, chances are you would work that limb more than the others to increase its strength – maybe even making that limb stronger than the others eventually. However, no matter how hard you train or work that limb, you will always be aware of an underlying weakness for which you are compensating.

Mars and the Body

Mars rules the nerve tissue, which has its origin in the bone marrow. It rules the haemoglobin in the blood, the liver, spleen, gallbladder, bile, uterus, head and eyebrows. Parasara describes Mars as 'cruel, has blood-red eyes, is fickle-minded, liberal-hearted, bilious and has a thin waist and thin physique'. Mars represents courage and sports as well as cuts, wounds, weapons and surgery. A strong Mars in the horoscope shows a strong energy, vigour and vitality. A weak, or afflicted Mars, shows problems with any of the tissues or organs mentioned as well as an overall lack of strength. In Ayurveda, Mars represents toxic heat in the body, leading to inflammation and its related illnesses. It also causes accidents. This is because when Mars is not expressed, the resulting build-up of tension needs an outlet that is usually experienced through anger being directed at others. This is then experienced as either anger being returned to you from others or by the experience of an accident.

When there is excessive heat in the body, it can lead to a need to control, such as a person or situation. This need expresses itself in the body as tension as the muscles tense in order to try and achieve some sense of control. This is no different when we exercise, where an individual strongly influenced by Mars would benefit by balancing fire in order to cool down this tendency of pushing too hard. Injuries are commonplace when Mars is looking for a healthy outlet it cannot find.

If you have a strong Mars in your horoscope, you may be very exacting and efficient, just as a surgeon needs to be exact with his or her incisions. Even being very logical is seen as a form of violence as there is a need to put a point across in a sharp and precise manner, leaving no room for debate. This is a build-up of heat and the controlling nature of Mars. In a healthy expression of the Mars impulse, an individual gets to the point and is logical without having to beat anyone over the head with a point of view. An unhealthy expression of Mars may show a person can either lack logic and make that person timid in expressing an opinion, or compensate by forcefully expressing a point of view. When anger is involved, fear is at its root as fire cannot exist without air.

The goal of Mars is to destroy anything that we perceive to be making us weak. This may be something physical, mental or emotional. Tuesday is a good day to use the energy of Mars and take on a task that requires courage and action with precision in order to achieve a personal goal. For someone with a strong Mars, it may not be necessary to strengthen this planet any further as this could lead to too much aggression. However, for someone with a weak Mars, it may be necessary to strengthen a sense of personal power. This could be done through learning to be more assertive by taking on courses or routes that facilitate this. In general, having a strong will and ambition can lead one into too much risk taking at times.

Exercise for Mars

Any exercise for Mars would ideally incorporate a more dynamic approach to movement. This type of exercise could be used any time you feel irritable and angry. Ultimately, exercise should aim to restore balance and calm by cooling down and allowing things to gradually unfold as they need to. As Mars energy needs a target, it may be more beneficial to give yourself a more balanced end result as your aim. Any exercise would ideally begin with a warm-up that leads to a more vigorous workout, facilitating the Mars need to achieve and an impulse to fight. Exercises that are deemed to be too strenuous could be left out as this would only increase your push and drive into a state of imbalance. If there is tension or irritability, then you already are experiencing an imbalance. You should always be aware of pushing too hard and causing injury when

Mars is strongly influencing. If you feel your breath becoming too laboured, then this is an indication of pushing too hard, in which case it would be more beneficial to rest in order to regain balance.

Exercise should gradually become more restorative and allowing. This encourages the natural flow of life to occur and has a knock-on effect on your day. You may think of this as pre-paving your day, which saves you a lot of energy in the long run. Most strongly Mars-influenced individuals think that life requires a lot more physical energy to achieve results than is actually necessary. This is a poor expression of Mars' other talents, one of which is the willpower to achieve a goal by simply focusing your intention and attention. Many athletes visualise an achievement before committing themselves to it physically. However, visualisation alone does not express Mars to the fullest. Without some physical expression, you would find the energy building into an uncontrollable urge to do something. This should not be an all-or-nothing approach as it can be with a 'Mars-type'. Do what needs to be done and then just allow it to be. Getting this balance of doing and being is one of the most rewarding aspects of an exercise programme and one that benefits the Mars impulse enormously.

Aries and Scorpio – Embodying Mars

If either Aries or Scorpio is your rising sign, then Mars takes on a powerful role for you. To see how you express this important destructive impulse, look to its placement in your chart. Mars, like any planet, will gain greatly from being in its own sign (Aries or Scorpio) or in its exaltation sign, Capricorn. The Mars impulse is well suited to the hard-working sign Capricorn, where we can apply a disciplined approach to achieve whatever we perceive to strengthen us. It is debilitated in the opposite sign of Cancer, where it does not feel so comfortable in dealing with the emotional issues of the Moon, which requires that one's feelings in the moment dictate actions. This position can lead to frustration and a lack of personal drive, often giving into other's needs or avoiding what needs to be done based on how one feels.

If you have the sign Aries or Scorpio as your rising sign, you are an embodiment of Mars and this energy will need some form of expression on a daily basis in order to avoid a build-up of tension. The aforementioned need to control will result if there is no outlet for Mars. Aries will do so more openly as it is an assertive, masculine sign. Scorpio will do so more passively (or passive aggressively!) as it is Mars' feminine sign. Look to see where Mars is placed in your horoscope by house position in order to see where you like to take action in your life.

Mercury

Mercury represents the intellect, speech, education and travel. It shows how we communicate so all forms of communication come under its domain. It is commonly pictured as the winged messenger, taking messages back and forth from the soul to us here on Earth as it transits between the Earth and the Sun. It is seen as a fickle planet, being easily influenced by whatever it associates with in the horoscope. Those who are strongly influenced by Mercury will exhibit the same attributes. Its state in the chart is therefore dependent on its associations with other planets. This can make the planet, though naturally a benevolent energy, become more malevolent when associating with any of the naturally malevolent planets. Though this is true to some degree of any of the planets, this is never more relevant as it is in the case of Mercury.

Think of a computer screen. The screen will bring up any information you ask it to. That is the ability of the mind. We must be aware of what we are subjecting the screen of our minds to and whether this is a positive or negative influence. The true strength of Mercury is one of discrimination – being able to ascertain a right course of action in our exercise routines, for example. Our analytical minds like to gather lots of facts and figures, representing our reasoning capacity. It is through this process that we become skilled in anything worldly as Mercury represents the densest and most practical element of earth. Earth has all of the elements in life's building blocks. By developing life skills, we develop an ability to work and interact with others in the world.

If Mercury is well placed in the horoscope, it will manifest as an intellectual, witty and also, perhaps, a fickle type of individual. We can see how our modern world has a predominance of Mercurial energy as expressed in an age of too much information that we need to process constantly. In this way, we can see Mercury and Mercurial-type people having to always work things out using the intellect.

Do not expect Mercury types to be truthful with you always. Sometimes this might not even be a deliberate deception, but in any case, when the mind is working out the many possibilities on any given topic, there is always room to manoeuvre. Mercury-type individuals may even be said to be two-faced because of this. If Mercury is strongly placed to represent your nature, then it can show a person of an excitable and nervous nature. Radio broadcasters need to have Mercury strongly influencing them in order to be able to maintain a witty repertoire throughout a broadcast.

Mercury and the Body

Mercury is appropriately seen as having the attributes of all three humours. It takes on the attributes of the planets it becomes influenced by in relation to the humours. For example, if Mercury is placed with Mars, the mind becomes more logical and can express impatience, taking on a more argumentative stance. Mercury rules the dual signs of Gemini and Virgo, which further points towards the mind's dual nature. Mercury rules the plasma, hips, skin, forehead, throat, mouth and tongue. Any afflictions to Mercury will bring up issues in relation to these areas. Parasara's description of Mercury is that he 'possesses an attractive physique ... He has a blend of all three humours of bile, phlegm and wind.'

Exercise for Mercury

Any exercise for Mercury would ideally be geared to quietening down a busy mind, while integrating all that one has learned. Technique-based exercises may supply the intellectual requirements a Mercury type has in order to do something more beneficial with the impulse than needless gossip and irrelevant information. Mercury types always need something for the mind to chew over. Team sports that require dexterity and lots of interaction between players can facilitate this need.

Ultimately, the goal would be to quieten down the mind and delve into an inner intelligence that we have access to once the mind is still. This is where there is no need to work things out on an intellectual level. It may be more beneficial to gain access to a teacher so that he or she can teach you techniques without too much intellectual stimulation on your part. Too much intellectual stimulation keeps the mind engaged at a superficial level only.

Gemini and Virgo – Embodying Mercury

If Gemini or Virgo is your rising sign, then Mercury takes on the role of expressing your nature. Mercury, being a changeable and impressionable planet, shows that wherever it goes, it will take on the attributes of that planet. It is, therefore, important to surround yourself with those who will encourage you to continue in whatever exercise routines balance you. Mercury finds its masculine, more assertive expression through the air-dominant sign Gemini. Gemini, though a masculine sign, is represented by a male and female, sometimes depicted as twins (male and female), sometimes as lovers. This hints at the duality of Mercury and the propensity to play with different points of view and perspectives. This can occur without the need to arrive at any definite conclusions that can waste a lot of energy on debate. The portion of the body that Gemini represents is the neck, arms and hands, showing this tendency to look around and pick and choose from a variety of options. However, if there are too many choices on offer, such as too many ways of working with the body, there may be a lack of achievement in preference for a good debate. The other indication of the sign Gemini is of interaction and flirtation. The Sanskrit name for Gemini, *Mithuna*, derives from *Maithuna*, literally translated as 'sexual intercourse'. Mercury enjoys playing with words and with sexuality as it is a neuter planet, which again points to the masculine and feminine achieving a balanced state.

Mercury finds its more feminine expression through the sign Virgo, where practical concerns are prominent. Here Mercury finds its expression through working things out in order to calculate the risks and eliminate anything that is counterproductive. The sign Virgo is where we have this ability to pick apart all that is not required for assimilation. Any individual with this sign rising will have this innate capacity and expertise. Mercury is exalted in its earth-dominant sign of Virgo, where it likes to deal with the practicalities of life. It is debilitated in the water-dominant sign Pisces, where it feels out of its depth in such a formless realm. Virgo, being a very analytical sign and dominant in the earth element, suits the energy of Mercury, which rules the earth element. Pisces is the water-dominant sign of the priestly Jupiter and Mercury cares little for the more emotional and religious aspects of life. Jupiter is the teacher and has lots to teach the student Mercury, but he may not always want the deeper lessons and may spend hours in debate and conjecture. This represents the relationship our own intuition (Jupiter) has with our more rational concerns (Mercury). Though you may know something to be true deep down, you may engage in a lot of discourse to convince your intellect of such an intuition. You may know that a certain exercise or movement is not appropriate for you, but you may have to study why this is so before you satisfy the Mercurial impulse. Look to see the house position of Mercury in your horoscope in order to ascertain where you like to engage your intellect and apply what you have learned.

Jupiter

Jupiter represents the wisdom we gain from life experience. It represents teachers, advisers, wise counsel and the good fortune we are due based on previous right thoughts, words and actions. Jupiter is the largest planet in our solar system and because of its expansive nature it can bring growth to whatever area of the chart it is focused upon. This may mean to your physical body also. If it is placed in your first house, then it can mean it will give you a larger body, not taking into account any other indications.

Jupiter represents advisers who offer wise counsel. It also represents the ability to listen and be guided. If you have a strong Jupiter in your chart, then chances are you have a strong inner guidance (intuition) that will be of benefit to you and will help you make the right decisions in any course of action. A weakly placed Jupiter shows a lack in the ability to tune into this inner guidance as well as a lack of faith. Jupiter holds things and people together as it rules the element of space, which contains and organises all of the elements. If someone has a very strong Jupiter influencing them, they will have the capacity to organise large groups of people and hold a space for them. This is one of the roles of a teacher. However, if Jupiter is weakly placed, there may be issues around organising others or even organising one's own life, whether this is with regards to an exercise routine or any daily practice.

Jupiter and the Body

According to Parasara, Jupiter 'is large bodied, has honey coloured eyes and hair, is phlegmatic...' Jupiter rules the fat tissue, belly, liver, spleen, gallbladder, pancreas and ears. The colours of Jupiter are yellow and gold. It rules Thursday and so this is a good day to expand your life in some way. This may be achieved by being guided by a teacher. This may also take the form of travel or study of any kind. Jupiter represents an inner intelligence, which does not need the input of the intellect.

Exercise for Jupiter

Any exercise routine for Jupiter could be accentuated or begun on a Thursday. Exercise can be used to tune into your inner guide when a particular situation needs your deeper awareness. Letting the body's inner intelligence guide you in your movement will help you tune into the strength of Jupiter. No matter what a class environment or teacher's guidance may dictate, if you feel a stronger nudge towards a particular course of action, then listen to that inner wisdom above anyone else. You may need to seek out a teacher, guide or instructor if this is not something you feel able to connect with. The ultimate goal is to develop your own inner intelligence in any movement-based activities you perform.

Exercise to uplifting music and make sure to allow the awareness to rest on the spaces between the breaths. This is an instant way of tuning into the inner voice that is always present. Sometimes keeping the space free from as much external noise as possible will help this process if it is not a natural state for you. Even if there is noise, you can always tune into the cosmic hum that is always reassuringly present.

Sagittarius and Pisces – Embodying Jupiter

If Sagittarius or Pisces is your rising sign, then you are an embodiment of Jupiter. When Jupiter takes on this role, it shows a very idealistic individual. Look to see where Jupiter is placed by house position and how this is tempered by the qualities of the sign. Look to see if Jupiter is placed in an inert, active or harmonious sign as well as the dominant element of the sign.

Jupiter is exalted in the sign of Cancer and debilitated in the sign opposite in Capricorn. In Cancer, Jupiter finds the realm of care and sustenance of the home and community of the utmost importance, as Jupiter represents the part of our being that is chiefly concerned with upholding the natural laws – following a tradition, doing something the way it has always been done. Practices such as yoga and martial arts may be ways of following a well-worn path that is easy to navigate due to the guidance of others who have gone before you.

Jupiter is weakest in Capricorn as it has to deal with, but has no time for, the everyday practicalities of life and its harsh realities. In Capricorn, there is no time for the high moral ground, as well as a more optimistic outlook of a strong Jupiter. In Capricorn, there is the reality of living a practical life, which may leave little room for the more profound experiences Jupiter can offer us. Look to see where Jupiter is placed in your horoscope by house position in order to connect with what gives meaning to your life.

Venus

Venus represents the pleasant things in life, such as sex, physical comforts, a social life, enjoyment of food, clothes, the arts and entertainment. Its placement will show how one expresses love and affection, and the way in which one goes about finding love and affection from others. For both men and women, it rules married life; but, more specifically, it represents women in the horoscope. Venus rules Friday, making it a good day to seek some enjoyment in life, whether by enjoying the arts or simply your own company and surroundings. The things in life that bring us happiness are represented by

Venus and these will depend on the position and strength of Venus in the chart. The entertainment and fashion industries come under the domain of Venus and, depending on where you have Venus placed in your chart, will show how you express your own sense of style. The colour for Venus is not one single colour but multi-coloured, like the light being shone through a diamond (a Venus gemstone), creating a prism of colours.

If you have a weak Venus in your horoscope, you may have difficulty expressing yourself as a sexual being and be uncomfortable when it comes to how you present yourself aesthetically. If Venus is afflicted in your chart, there may be issues around your expression of the sexual urge and perversions may be a result. If you have a strong Venus and it has an aspect on, or rules your first house, then you should have no problem expressing yourself as a sexual being and can easily dress up for any occasion. Charming your way around a room should come easy as Venus can smooth over the rough edges of life. The highest form of love, as seen by Venus exalted in Pisces, is unconditional love and devotion. Venus is in debility in Virgo, which is ruled by the practical Mercury and is the sign of virtue, a domain Venus does not like to find itself in. Venus in Virgo does not express itself very well because of the need for perfection in this sign, and because it is the natural 6th house of the zodiac, dealing with everyday drudgery. In our relationships, such perfection and nit-picking does not lend itself to a harmonious relationship. There may be sexual enjoyment when Venus is in Virgo, but when Venus is weakly placed it is looking for love in all the wrong places. Our highest expression of Venus is unconditional love and when we cannot access that, we will seek it everywhere else, hoping to satisfy our desires. When it is at its strongest, there is a sense of happiness regardless of the situation, whereas when it is weak, we seek to always find the perfect situation that will make us happy.

Venus rules the water element so it is seen as a harmonising presence in the horoscope by virtue of the water smoothing over all of life's rough edges and balancing our hormones and water content in the body. Without Venus, life would become too harsh and dry, so we need to accentuate this quality in our lives if we wish to make it more pleasurable. However, if we overindulge Venus, we can end up feeling lazy and lack the motivation to better ourselves in physical activities.

Venus and the Body

Venus rules the reproductive fluid, the face and eyes, the kidneys, the endocrine and urinary systems, and the reproductive organs. When there is a severe malefic influence to the planet, there can be difficulty in any of these areas. Venus has an excess of air and water in its constitution and, according to Parasara, 'is joyful, charming in physique, has beautiful eyes ... is phlegmatic and windy and has curly hair'.

Exercise for Venus

Exercise with Venus in mind can be cultivated on a Friday, or when the need for a more comfortable experience arises. Learn to love your routine and enjoy the experience of being in your body. Allow the body to find the balance it is always gravitating towards with ease. Comfort and happiness are the positive expressions of Venus, which can find an outlet through a more fluid, fun-filled exercise routine – perhaps enjoying the company of others while you exercise. Dance is one such expression of Venus in action. Enjoy the sensuality of your body and the pleasure it provides you. Try not to luxuriate in it too much, however, as this can increase laziness, one of Venus' more negative attributes. Instead, you can seek balance between comfort and effort, which facilitate each other, and find a happy medium.

Libra and Taurus – Embodying Venus

If you have Taurus or Libra as your rising sign, then Venus becomes an important planet in your constitutional makeup. Your nature is coloured greatly by your need for love and harmony. This may mean you needing to express yourself through the mirror of another and to find balance in relationships, or perhaps in the balance of colours and words, as seen in many artistic expressions. The particular quality of your artistic expression and needs in love will be seen by the sign position of Venus. When Venus is placed in Mars' signs, there is usually a more pronounced physical expression in art, such as in dance. A fire sign like Aries will show a go-getter and a passionate disposition. Look to see where you apply Venus qualities by its house placement as this shows where you like to experience pleasure. If Venus is placed in your first house, then you are no doubt a pleasure-seeker.

Saturn

With time, we learn how to discipline ourselves and realise that those bad habits no longer serve us and instead make us ill. Having a strong, unaffected Saturn in the horoscope will show someone who has the ability to discipline themselves in a daily workout routine. Saturn teaches us to work hard, but not to have any attachment to an end result. This approach helps us greatly because if we are always looking for a result, we get discouraged for most of the time we are working towards it. Until we eventually arrive at our goal, we are not at our goal. So the lesson Saturn teaches us is patience. It represents all of the hard lessons we have to learn when applied to any area of our life, but in exercise Saturn teaches us restraint and responsible practices.

Saturn represents sorrow, limitations, restrictions and delays, and is the planet of difficulties, which cannot be avoided. We have debts to clear that are based on our past thoughts, words and actions, and because of this, Saturn represents the debt that needs to be repaid. Saturn's placement will show the areas of life in which we have to pay back these debts. This is true at birth and changes with the passage of time. This is seen by observing the transits of Saturn with the aid of an astrologer or astrology resource, as we continue making choices that are either going to yield positive or negative results for the future.

Saturn can bring hardships to us because of wrong thinking, and can also make us somewhat melancholic or even depressed, especially if it has an association with the Moon in the horoscope. Because of its restricting effect, when Saturn transits or aspects a certain planet in your chart, it slows that area down. For example, when it transits or aspects your first house or your first house ruling planet, it can be a time to pay particular attention to your body. It may be a time to slow down and pay attention to your health and what you are doing to improve yourself.

If you have a strong Saturn in your horoscope (placed in exaltation in Libra, its own signs Capricorn or Aquarius, or in a friendly environment in Mercury and Venus signs), it can mean you can take on the responsibility that Saturn is asking of you. If Saturn is weak in your chart (placed in debilitation in Aries, or in the Sun, Moon, Mars or Jupiter signs), it may mean you have difficulty facing up to life's challenges. Someone who is defined as a 'Saturn-type' could be described as responsible, if somewhat serious. The darkness of Saturn (Saturn is the farthest planet from the Earth observable to the naked eye) needs to be balanced with the light of the Sun. So if you are experiencing Saturn strongly, it would be beneficial to bring in some light, either in the form of actual sunlight, a comedy, a sun food diet, or indeed studying *Jyotish*, the 'science of light'.

I have noted in my astrology consultations over the years that many clients take to a yoga and meditation practice in a Saturn time period. There are a number of reasons for this. One is that we experience pain in a Saturn period and we seek to alleviate this pain, whether it is physical, mental or emotional. This is a lot of people's introduction to yoga and its healing benefits. Another reason many begin the path of yoga during a Saturn period is that the planet represents the air element and we begin to experience the effects of air. This can be felt as separation, loneliness and isolation that can lead to fear and depression or it can be experienced as a joyful detachment that is felt in meditation. Being alone with others in a yoga class or meditation group gives us a sense of the space we are all held in. This is because air is contained within space. One way we can access space is through the breath. Every time we acknowledge the breath, we are acknowledging Saturn. However, this must be balanced with acknowledging the spaces between breaths in order to counteract the tendency to be too time-focused and stressed out as a result.

Another reason why working with the path of yoga, or any type of physical work or activity, suits a Saturn time period is that Saturn represents the muscle tissue. We work the muscles when we exercise, of course, ideally without any sense of gain from what we are doing. It should be done for the work itself in the moment. It can bring us into the moment by bringing us into our bodies and our breath. We learn to let go eventually and can relax the body completely as we rest at the end of a workout. This is an expression of Saturn every day in an exercise routine, and the more we can express this, the less we have to experience the negative effects of Saturn otherwise. Body-builders are very 'Saturn-type' individuals. They work hard on their musculature in a committed and consistent manner. However, this must be balanced with a strong Mars impulse, which controls the nerves in any executed movement.

The Lord of Time

Saturn gives us a sense of time, being the Lord of time, structure and form. We become so aware of the choices we have made and the results of those choices that we can be paralysed with fear, not wishing to create any more negativity for ourselves. This inert aspect of Saturn holds us back through fear as we begin to limit our movement, whether mentally, emotionally or physically. We must move through this fear, ultimately, and let go of anything that is holding us back. Once we learn to let go of old baggage, we can then move on feeling lighter – just as a detox benefits us by making us feel lighter afterwards. It may be painful while we detox, but the rewards are great afterwards. It may also be painful to maintain a physical exercise regime at times, but we know that the rewards are great if we stay the course in a consistent and responsible manner.

Saturn is exalted in Libra and debilitated in Aries. It rules the signs Capricorn and Aquarius, and anyone with either one of these as their rising sign may be described as somewhat serious. There is, at the very least, a drive to achieve something. This is because when Saturn is strong, it represents hard work, discipline, focus, consistency and determination – all the qualities it takes to see something through with time. Time it will take, no doubt, as Saturn is the slowest-moving planet and will slow everything down for us to pay attention. If Saturn is weak in the horoscope, then a lack of these more positive qualities will show up as fear, doubt, guilt, shame, laziness and slothfulness – all the qualities of inertia. Even a strong Saturn will express some of these at different times, as is the nature of this slow-moving planet. The very necessary limitation of Saturn allows us to move forward eventually in whatever course of action we take. We must, however, work within the limits of our being. Just as we need lines in the road to safely reach our destination, we need the order of Saturn to keep us in line.

Saturn and the Body

Saturn represents the muscle tissue, thighs, colon, rectum, knees, legs and joints. In Ayurvedic terms, it is seen as inert air and causes most diseases. Ayurveda has 80 classifications of disease for the air humour, only 40 for the fire humour and 20 for the water humour. Saturn being the primary planet of air confirms its role in health-related issues. Parasara describes Saturn as having 'an emaciated and long physique, honey coloured eyes, is windy in temperament, has big teeth … lame and coarse, rough hair'.

Look to see where Saturn is placed in your chart by sign and by house position as these are areas you may have to experience some illness on some level – be it physical, mental or emotional. This will be more relevant during a Saturn period. The best way to approach Saturn is on your knees. Becoming humble is the strength of Saturn, but this result often necessitates being humiliated. Work hard in the areas of your life that Saturn represents. As it moves around the different parts of our life by transit, we may have to learn the lesson of detachment as people and things are removed or denied in our life experience. The ultimate goal of Saturn is that we learn to become detached and more spiritually aware. When everything has been taken away from us, then what else is there to turn to? Saturn represents the very real issues we deal with in life, but in doing so, it points us to the very real experience of our true spiritual essence.

We all know that if we lived a responsible life and worked hard at every area of our being, then we would have no negative repercussions as a result. Of course, we do not always do that, so the placement of Saturn will show where we can work hard now as we build again from the ruins of our past mistakes. The qualities of consistency and responsibility are not always present when we are young; but, like the image of old-man Saturn, we become more and more like him as we age.

As we grow older, air increases and we begin to dry out, showing our ability to detach from life. If we are unable to access this detachment, there can be fear at losing everything. Yet, we all know we will lose everyone and everything eventually. This is a necessary part of living in a physical body, represented by the process of death and decay. This detachment can be developed sooner than later so we do not have to experience the negative effects of this inevitable loss. We can take on the task of working without any self-interest and benefit from our hard work. This becomes easier the more we have taken away as, if and when we receive a bounty in our lives again; we no longer view it in the same way. We realise that everything and everyone will be taken away from us at some point. We do not just intellectualise this process after a loss in our lives, but instead we feel what that is like and we bow in humility and defeat to the Lord of Time, Saturn.

Exercise for Saturn

Any exercise for Saturn is beneficial and could be accentuated or begun on a Saturday. The emphasis could be more on a detoxifying set of routines or exercises, with the goal of feeling lighter afterwards. This lightness can then be brought into your day and is a good way to experience a sense of detachment in your life. Stay with routines for longer periods as you build resilience – another product of Saturn's influence. Any activity where you are strongly engaging the muscles and/or focusing on the breath will be beneficial in appeasing the influences of Saturn. Saturn represents the impulse to flee from danger whether one actually moves the body or not. So it may be more beneficial to use the energy which would ordinarily be put into fleeing in order to reduce the stress felt by this response.

Fasting on Saturn's Day

A fast is a great practice to cultivate on a Saturday – Saturn's day. It clears the body of toxins, leaving you feeling lighter and clearer, reducing dullness. If you do it with a sense of appeasing the energy of Saturn in your life, then the practice takes on a deeper dimension. Your body begins to look forward to the rest it receives every week, and if you experience the limitation of not eating for just one day a week, you will not have to experience as much of the negative effects of Saturn otherwise. You are purposefully inviting the experience of limitation into your life.

The clearing process of Saturn can be a painful one, just as a detox can make you feel uncomfortable at times, but ultimately you know you will benefit from it. This is the same whether you fast physically, mentally or emotionally. You may wish to meditate in a formal practice of meditation or in a more meditative experience of movement through exercise in order to observe the negative thoughts you think, the negative emotions you feel – letting them all pass through you and out. You are not suppressing these thoughts and emotions, yet you are not fixated on them, either. We can often experience the dulling effect of Saturn and the resulting toxicity by thinking more negatively or by trying to avoid feeling anything at all. We must experience whatever feelings are looking for expression, allowing them to come up and letting them go. A meditation practice can facilitate this as can an exercise routine. We observe negative thought patterns and prevent them from taking too firm a hold. While moving the body, we move the negative emotions through us. Balance and harmony are a result of this process. Observing the breath is a crucial part of this experience as it brings us into the present moment and into our bodies during the whole process. With a Saturn experience, we are all too often not present, experiencing sadness when we are stuck in the past or fear while projected into the future.

The tendency of a Saturn experience is to become so aware of space and time that we are no longer in our bodies. We observe the difficulties we are facing in a Saturn period and realise they are the results of wrong choices made previously, which brings us into the past. We also become intensely aware of the choices we are currently making in creating our future, which also keeps us from being fully in the present moment. Observing this tendency in any activity is a need to balance these tendencies as we come into the breath and the present moment in our bodies in exercise.

When we observe the space between breaths, we have gone deeper still, acknowledging the space on a deeper and more subtle level of our being. We are literally given space to breathe. The awareness of form (our separate bodies and life experience) and time (consequences of choices we make) all can hold us back in fear. The role of Saturn is to allow us to experience being separate with our own needs, which are important. However, if we let this become the only experience we have in life, it can be completely isolating. The fear, though protecting us from danger, can take over our lives and we can fear everything and everyone. So spend time with others in activities that are uplifting and fun to perform, as opposed to always having to work hard on yourself and your chosen discipline.

Capricorn and Aquarius – Embodying Saturn

If either Capricorn or Aquarius is your rising sign, then look to see where and how you apply the impulse of Saturn in your life. Wherever Saturn and these signs are placed in your horoscope shows where you feel insecure to some degree or other. For those with Saturn ruling their first house, there can be issues around shining their light in the world. This lends itself to stepping back and allowing others to shine while you do the ground work for them.

The Lunar Nodes – Rahu & Ketu

The nodes of the Moon, which represent the eclipses, are not physical bodies – they are shadows. Therefore, it is difficult to tell how their effects will manifest in our lives. This is the obscuring influence of the eclipses. The nodes are greatly influenced by the planets they associate with and by where they are positioned in the horoscope, exaggerating whatever they have an influence on – just as shadows obscure and exaggerate whatever they influence. The changes that the nodes bring about can be said to be that of a psychological nature, but ultimately this change occurs in every area of our lives as we evolve beyond where we are. There can be a huge internal churning effect and outward changes in the way we perceive things. This churning effect can be one where we deal with our inner demons and bring up some unpleasant things to experience, but we can also gain some insights and deal with things in a more innovative way as a result. This leads us to make jumps in our evolution as human beings.

The north and south nodes are always obscuring the Sun and Moon, and it is because of these points in the horoscope that we experience eclipses. Think of what happens when there is an eclipse. The light of the Sun or Moon is temporarily obscured so that we get the opportunity to see into the depths of space. The eclipses offer us the opportunity to view things differently, though this experience brings with it all kinds of irrational fears – as is the nature of shadows. When we are dealing with shadows, they can be a difficult territory for us to navigate. They can bring up all kinds of obsessions and compulsions, disturbing the mind. The insights during an eclipse or in their time period can have a profound effect on us.

Though both the north and south nodes are looked at separately to show influences on both ends of the spectrum, they are both part of a whole and need to be studied as such. The north node represents the soul's need to achieve and propels us forward, creating new experiences for ourselves. The south node represents the soul's past and the need to let go of outworn ways of being, creating disillusionment in our present state of being.

Rahu – The North Node

Wherever the north node sits in your horoscope shows where the soul is coming into this life with no experience and where we have an insatiable thirst for life experience. This also comes with a sense of inadequacy. It is in these areas of our lives that we find our needs are never fulfilled. No matter how much is achieved in these areas, it can give us a sense of never really having fully digested the experience. This would be more prevalent in periods of the north node. It represents all things foreign and unusual, where we do things differently and can be obsessive and compulsive in this area of our life.

The North Node and the Body

In Ayurvedic terms, the north node is seen as toxic air, just like Saturn. It is likened to Saturn in many ways, both representing the air element. However, the north node shows a distortion of air and can create many disturbances because of this. If Saturn is the separation we feel in our lives because of air, then the north node is that air being whipped up into a frenzy. We have no grounding in a reality from which to relate to others. That is why in a time period of the north node, we are less grounded and in touch with others. During a north node experience, it is important to exercise the body in order to remain grounded. We may become isolated during a north node time period, but we must not lose sight of others and their needs also. It can, however, lead to all kinds of insights and innovations in our routines and ways of performing actions when we are not so influenced by how others are performing such actions.

The north node represents the hands, mouth, lips, ears and extrasensory functions. It can bring disturbances that cannot be easily understood or treated as it is not a planet and, as such, is hard to define and cure as a result. Parasara describes the north node, along with the south node, as having a 'blue body ... is windy in temperament ...' Because of its co-rulership of Aquarius alongside Saturn, you can look to see which area (house position) Aquarius represents in your horoscope. Look to see the house and sign position of the north node in your horoscope. This will be indicated by *Rahu* – the Sanskrit name for the north node of the Moon. This will give you an idea of where you feel this urgency to achieve something in life, but where you may also experience compulsions that drive you away from ever being completely satisfied. If it sits in your first house, then you may never be satisfied with yourself as you continually try to improve yourself through different means. It is important to balance this tendency with simply being happy with where you find yourself, be it in your fitness goals or your competitive targets.

Exercise for the North Node

For a north node-influenced exercise programme, you would ideally keep your environment free from artificial influences as much as possible. Make sure it is free from any technology or any disturbances of any kind related to technology. If you are strongly influenced by the north node, then you would ideally create a more natural and more organised environment in which to exercise. This impulse represents the unusual so to take some of this on board, you could add something of the unusual to the setting. For most of us here in the West, the practice of yoga, for example, adds this element as it is not usually something we have been brought up with from birth. You could also exercise in a way you have never exercised before or simply discover a new way of doing something you have never thought of before. Every time you engage with whatever feels unusual or innovative to you, you are engaging this type of quality.

The north node, representing a disturbance of air, can be experienced by always being in the future, plotting, scheming and generally not being very present. Any exercise should address this tendency. Some may be more geared towards thrill-seeking activities that take you to the edge and into the present moment. Be generous to yourself by simply allowing space to be, instead of always needing to achieve something extreme.

Aquarius – Embodying the North Node

Embodying the north node seems like a misdemeanour as Rahu is seen as a head without a body in Vedic myth! It is ungrounded and creates desires that raise their compulsive heads during its period, and in relation to its position in the horoscope. If Aquarius is your rising sign, then the north node takes on an important role along with the planet Saturn. This combines the seriousness of Saturn with the unorthodox approach of the north node. Both create detachment and aloofness in an Aquarius individual. However, this detachment allows an Aquarius individual to be of the greatest assistance in society by observing things from afar and with great ingenuity. See where the north node (Rahu) is placed by house placement as this shows the area you experience a taste for the unusual. This is the very nature of air and of air types, who find change blowing in constantly.

Ketu – The South Node

The south node represents the past and shows what you are willing to give up. Past life connections can be studied from the south node's position in the horoscope. This is, however, only useful if it is helpful in your present context. The south node connects us to the past and our baggage while the north node connects us to the future and our need to create more. It is important to note that they are both part of a whole. They represent our sense of separation from this sense of wholeness, driving us forward into new situations and looking back at previous ones, albeit subconsciously. In the mythical story of how they were created, the outcast demon *Vasuki* drank of Amrita (immortal nectar) and thus became immortal. He had deceived the Gods to obtain the nectar and his head was cut off for this deceit. In this way, *Rahu* became the head of the demon and *Ketu*, the headless body – the south node of the Moon.

One way to see which is influencing you more at any time is to ask yourself this question: If everyone you know were to disown you, would you stomp around and try and cause as much chaos as possible, making a show of yourself (north node), or would you say that you do not need anyone anyway and retreat into your own secluded world (south node)?

The south node connects to the unusual, just like the north node. However, the south node's influence removes things from our lives. This is a good thing if these things are bad habits and routines. It can tune us into secret knowledge and give us access to the past where we can tap into a wealth of experience from which we can draw strength.

The South Node and the Body

Parasara describes the south node in the same way he describes the north node. However, they exist on opposite ends of the colour spectrum. The north node represents ultra-violet on the colour spectrum; the south node represents infra-red. The south node is usually considered reddish in appearance by most Vedic astrologers because of this. It is seen as representing toxic heat in the same vein as Mars. However, the results can be harder to predict, owing to the hidden aspect of an eclipse. The south node causes illnesses that are difficult to treat. They are usually more intense in nature than 'Mars-type' illnesses. The south node represents the legs, hair and extrasensory functions.

Exercise for the South Node

Exercise with emphasis on clearing excessive heat would be beneficial, although the south node's nature is to work on a more psychological level. Just as with the north node, the south node also brings the element of the unusual into your life so if you are strongly influenced by this impulse, (having the south node in your first house, for example) then you may want to accentuate this in your exercise routines. Any hidden or occult knowledge that includes access to powerful transformative exercises would be beneficial in tapping into this impulse. The south node is represented by a headless body, showing a need to simply feel into our past through the body, as opposed to working it out in our head. As you delve deeply into your exercises, things may surface that seem unexpected or unusual to your sense of self. Perform activities with the intention of staying with the feelings, viewing them objectively. This advice may only resonate with those who are strongly influenced by a time period of the south node of the Moon, Ketu.

Scorpio – Embodying the South Node

If you have the sign Scorpio as your rising sign, then the south node takes on the role, along with Mars, of expressing your nature. The fact that the south is seen as headless shows that there is often an irrational expression and more often than not this is not expressed outwardly in Scorpio, the sign representing our secrets. This is often the case with those who have the sign Scorpio prominent in their horoscope. Look to see where the south node (Ketu) is in your horoscope. This can add heat into the mix. Ultimately, the impulse of the south node will transform this area as this is another indication of its co-rulership of the natural 8th house Scorpio, which relates to transformation. Whatever house position in which we have the south node will show where things are oftentimes hidden from even ourselves as we experience the effects of this placement as dissatisfaction in the material world. If the south node is placed in your first house, it can show a dissatisfaction with yourself, which drives you deeper and further into pursuits in order to find some sense of satisfaction.

CHAPTER 6 – VITAL SIGNS

Your Rising Sign

Knowing your rising sign is of great benefit to any exercise routine as it shows how you came into being. It is reflective of how you express yourself in your physical body. By witnessing this, you can then work with balancing any imbalances that may occur. The rising sign, as well as the ruling planet of this sign, is of huge importance to your exercise regime. Because we are always dealing with some imbalance or another – and an imbalance is usually expressed via an excess of an inherent energy –it becomes helpful to work with your natural tendencies by being able to counteract these tendencies with opposing qualities. If you are out of balance, then you will seek things that bring you further out of balance. Recognising your tendencies through your nature in the horoscope allows you to amend some of those imbalances. If, for example, an individual with the sign Aries as their rising sign (with no other strong indications to counteract the sign's tendencies) finds that they push themselves hard physically, more often than not the experience is of an imbalance, which is often experienced by having an injury. This need to push may, at times, bring a sense of balance if there is a state of inertia that needs to be worked through. Simply having the sign Aries as your rising sign will not indicate this always, as planets influence this sign, especially if there is a planet placed in the sign. The position of Saturn in Aries, for example, will ensure a more reserved individual who may benefit from a physically strong exercise programme, such as a steady and considered weight-training programme, in order to correct any imbalances and a tendency to suffer weakness physically. However, 'Aries-type' individuals generally benefit from a more conservative approach to exercise in order to counteract the aggressive tendencies of the sign.

Your rising sign shows how you came into the world when you were born and, therefore, how you initiate any activity. This is the sign that was rising on the east as you emerged from your mother's womb and shows the overall energy of your life, including (but not exclusive to) your temperament, physical body, health and confidence. The Vedic astrologer Visti Larsen writes in his book *Jyotish Fundamentals*, the rising sign 'is the most important ...' and one should make a final assessment using this sign for 'the native's basic and changeable nature, the predominant influences on his life, his health, strength, appearance, focus, spirituality and his intelligence'. Though this sign cannot be the only factor to examine in your approach to exercise, it is the best place to begin. When looking at the complexities of an individual's chart, it is clear to see that generalities only go so far to represent an individual. However, your rising sign will be very telling of how you feel in your body and how you initiate any activities.

Planets in Your Rising Sign

Any planet dominates where it is placed, though some do more so depending on the strength of the planet in that placement. As we are looking at your nature in terms of constitution, then any planet placed in the rising sign will dominate that area. If there are several planets placed therein, then the strongest will dominate. However, all of these planets will have an impact on your nature if placed in your rising sign.

If you have planets present, they will bring their energies into how you express yourself in life. You will find an expression for them to be able to express the impulse of the rising sign at birth. When you were born, the sign of the zodiac rising on the east shows how you came into being. It shows how you approach a situation in life and how you apply your intelligence to that situation. Finding a healthy expression for that in your life will be of great benefit. Adhering to what the planet in your first house, i.e., rising sign, is asking of you, will allow you to express the qualities of the rising sign with the aid of that planet.

The Sun in Your Rising Sign

The Sun in your rising sign will show someone who needs to shine. When the Sun is placed here, it brings great strength and vigour if it is strong and unobstructed. You will light up a room by your mere presence, and so you should. We all need to shine in whatever area the Sun is placed, i.e., the house in which it is placed as well as the house position of the Sun's sign, Leo. The Sun in your rising sign means that you were born around sunrise. The Sun energy does very well in such prominence in the first house of the horoscope. This will be tempered by its sign position, of course. For example, a person who is born with the Sun in the first house in debilitation, i.e., in Libra, will find it more of a challenge to express the solar qualities than someone who has the Sun in exaltation in Aries. Do not think of debilitation or exaltation as simply 'good' or 'bad', but instead think of it as everything is either good or bad for something. The Sun in debility in the first house can show an individual who can lead with humility.

The Moon in Your Rising Sign

The Moon in your rising sign will show you express a caring nature if the Moon is strong and unobstructed. How you go about this will depend on other factors. The nature of the Moon will change according to its sign position and its associations with other planets as well as being a continually changing phenomenon. Because it is the fastest-moving heavenly body, the Moon will show an ever-changing emotional landscape. The Moon is seen as the mother, the healer and carer. Some role that reflects the compassion of the Moon will be beneficial for you. If the Moon is full, then a water-dominant nature is expressed, whereas if it is new, then an air-dominant nature will need to be addressed. When approaching an exercise routine, the Moon's feeling-based considerations may outweigh the physical exercise concerns in the moment. It may be best to exercise when you feel like it as opposed to trying to set out a definite schedule of exercises and timings.

Mars in Your Rising Sign

Mars in your rising sign will bring an explosive tendency if you do not handle the energy well. Mars is an impulsive planet and can bring heat and a need to control. Arguments or, at the very least, irritability can be present if the energy of Mars is not facilitated. One way to facilitate this is to become more physically active in order to work out some of the heat through dynamic forms of exercise. Meditation is also a great way of cooling down the heat of Mars, but may not, in and of itself, express your more dynamic nature. No doubt you will have to come to terms with this impulsive nature and will need to find an outlet in some way or you will simply keep finding yourself in arguments with those around you. You will have a youthful appearance as is the nature of the youthful Mars, but may also be self-critical. This must be balanced with acceptance.

Mercury in Your Rising Sign

Mercury in your rising sign will show a curious nature. It shows someone who never rests easily because of a constant need for stimulation. This needs to find a healthy outlet in order to allow the mind to rest. One way to facilitate this is to study that which does not over-stimulate the intellect. However, this may not always satiate the ever-curious Mercurial nature and the need for new information all of the time. Today's society has an abundance of food for thought. It may help to turn off the TV and log off the Internet for some time. Apply your need for speed in studying a subject of value to you personally as opposed to frivolous and needless information and gossip. Mercury does express an adaptable nature that can easily be filtered through a flexible yoga practice, for example. Having Mercury in either the 1st, 5th or 9th house in the D-9 harmonic chart will show hatha yoga as a path for you also. Team sports or group activities may be a better use of your flirtatious nature with Mercury in your first house.

Jupiter in Your Rising Sign

Jupiter in your rising sign will show someone who has a more idealistic and philosophical approach to life. Needless gossip and chit-chat will not satisfy such an idealistic individual. Jupiter represents teachers, reflecting our own inner guidance, so finding your way to a teaching role might suit this prominent position for Jupiter. There is a need for expansion in some way in order to express your philosophies and ideas to others. On a physical level, this can show a water-type body and, because Jupiter is the largest of the planets, it can show a large body – either tall and sturdy or short and stocky. A daily exercise routine will keep the energy flowing and the ideas coming. Following a water-balancing approach to movement will help if this is your nature.

Venus in Your Rising Sign

Venus in the first house will show someone who likes to feel good. The expression is one of harmony and wanting to please others in order to achieve this, but make sure that this need does not become a way of forgoing your own needs to please others all of the time. Venus shows a love of the arts, so you will want to express this in a role that facilitates this. Feeling good in your physicality is one way this can be expressed. Luxuriate in a sense of comfort and peace in an exercise such as dance, for example, as you allow the body to balance itself effortlessly. Make sure not to overindulge, however, as this can be one of the expressions of Venus and the resulting laziness. Our pleasures benefit from a bit of restraint.

Saturn in Your Rising Sign

Saturn in the your rising sign will show someone who has the capability of feeling a sense of duty and a certain seriousness due to a sense of responsibility. This can be expressed in a disciplined and consistent daily exercise regime. Saturn is the worker of the planets and can lend itself to a focused and hard-working approach to life if it is strong in your chart. Be sure to lighten the seriousness with some cheer, seeing it as equally important to all of the hard work you carry out. Saturn is a hard task master and enables you to get the job done if it is well positioned in your horoscope. This quality lends itself to becoming more work-oriented – always seeking the truth of something whether it feels good or not. This quality can also be applied to a hard workout routine. Saturn is detached and somewhat aloof. With this planet in your first house, you may find yourself developing more of a solitary exercise routine, such as weight-lifting. Balance this need for isolation with spending time with others in a sport or class environment as this will give you the sense of support and connection with others. Any group work such as a yoga or fitness class can give you this sense of doing your own work with others who are also doing their own work.

The North Node in Your Rising Sign

When the north node is placed in your rising sign, there is a need to experience life in all of its many shades and variations. The influence is that of the unusual. This 'shadowy planet' is always moving backwards against the flow of the usual forward-moving planets, and the constant forward motion of the Sun and Moon. This lends itself to seeing and doing things differently. The north node represents something foreign and innovative, so finding expression through a routine that is unusual to your upbringing might be one way of expressing this impulse. Make sure not to overdo it as the north node makes you think big. If you feel like your need for experience and achievement is taking over, notice this and rein in your ambitions. The remedy for this is generosity. If you feel like you are becoming too ambitious, it is good to give time and energy to others. By helping others achieve that which you want yourself, you go a long way to achieving your own goals. This position lends itself to someone who may ask too much of themselves. It may be more beneficial to try the less-is-more approach now and then, simply being instead of always wishing to achieve something ground-breaking.

The South Node in Your Rising Sign

If the south node is in your rising sign, you will (just as with the north node) need to express your unusual nature. Seeing and doing things differently will be needs that have to be met in any physical activity. A routine that can facilitate this is, of course, beneficial as is the need to deepen the experience in whatever you choose. In the myth of Rahu and Ketu, Ketu became the headless body of the demon Vasuki. Ketu teaches us to let go of worldly attachments. A meditative routine that takes you more into your heart and body expresses this impulse. This is not always necessarily a rational experience. Balancing the two energies of the south and north nodes becomes prominent with either of these in your rising sign. As they are the eclipse points, having either of these in the rising sign will show a need to work with your shadow nature in whatever activities you choose.

The Qualities of the Signs

As we have observed earlier, signs are either masculine or feminine in nature as well as either fixed, movable or dual. However, each sign's ruling planet also has its innate nature, which is more inert, active or harmonious. This will result in an overall quality that may, or may not, be the sign's outward impulse. Though each of the four elements of air, fire, water and earth is represented by the signs, space is the element that contains all of the elements, so it influences all of the signs. Fire, for example, can find its expression through an active sign, as in the sign Aries, or in the harmonious sign Sagittarius.

The elements are either masculine or feminine. The air- and fire-dominant signs are more masculine, and the water- and earth-dominant signs are more feminine. I write 'more' masculine or feminine as each of the signs has an influence from each of the elements when broken down to their building blocks. This breakdown will not be covered in this book, but it is worth noting at this point. When reading that Aries is a fire-dominant sign, you should be aware that it has the influence of all of the building blocks of life and, therefore, all of the elements. However, it is dominant in the fire element and finds its expression through this element more comfortably. When a sign is more masculine in nature (as it is in the air- and fire-dominant signs), it has a more assertive quality that can be expressed in many different ways. The feminine signs (water- and earth-dominant signs) are more receptive in nature.

Whatever sign you have identified with, be it your rising, Moon or Sun sign, please take the time to read all of the signs to become more familiar with each of them. Note that we all experience all of the signs in different areas. Though your identity is largely tied up with and bound by the rising sign, it is only the beginning and should be treated as such. You may also pay attention to the sign in which your ruling planet sits as this will give you another layer of analysis and understanding of your unique nature when all of these factors are taken into account.

The Signs of the Zodiac

The following information on each rising sign can only be applied generally until looked at more specifically in your own horoscope. Planets placed in or influencing the sign, as well as the placement of the sign ruler, all give a truer picture of your constitution and temperament.

Aries – Embodying Mars' Masculine Nature

Aries is the natural first house of the zodiac and this alone is very telling of the initiating nature of your sign. If you have this sign as your rising, it will show an impulsive nature. You will have the ability to get things started and are capable of being pioneering in whatever field you choose as long as there is nothing holding you back. You have plenty of energy to do all that you wish to achieve and usually get it done.

Balancing Aries

Aries is an active, fire-dominant and masculine sign. There is a lot of outward moving energy as a result, but the possibility of achieving all that you set out to is pronounced. This outward drive will have to be met in an exercise regime. The best way to meet it is to first allow an expression of it and to then balance this with a more relaxed and allowing approach. As it is a fire-dominant sign and is ruled by the fiery planet Mars, there is a fire-dominant nature. If there are no other indications from other planets, i.e., planets in the sign, then all of the advice for balancing fire applies here. Mars is the part of our being that does not like to think – it just likes to take action. The best way to approach any activity is to facilitate the need for physical expression initially in order to quieten and cool the 'Mars-type' tendency to overheat and over-extend, which will only end in an injury of some kind at some time or another.

The end goal should be to gradually soften and allow things to happen in any activity as opposed to pushing past comfort zones all the time. Some effort is required, of course, but if that is all you bring to the table, then you will not come away feeling balanced. An exercise routine can fire up an Aries-type like nothing else. This may be high-velocity dangerous sports or any activity in which precision is required. You are an embodiment of the warrior planet Mars and it may help to think of the warrior in you as you step onto a yoga mat, a gym floor or into a pair of ski boots. Find a way that expresses the destructive impulse of a warrior in order to rid your life of people and habits that weaken you. However, try to cultivate more kindness towards yourself and others, noticing your need to compete in a class situation. You may use that competitiveness in order to find the motivation to continue with your routine, but try not to let it take over the reasons you are exercising in the first place. Ultimately, the only competition is with one's self.

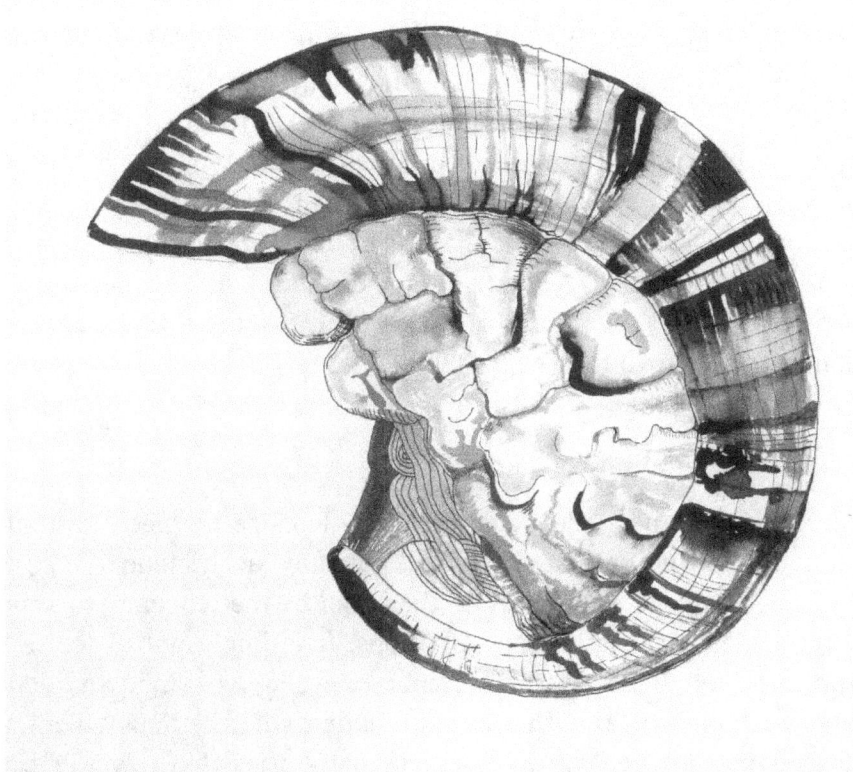

Aries Body Parts

Aries rules the head (back of the head and forehead). The symbol of Aries is the ram and your sign has a tendency to plough ahead without much consideration or forethought. Give yourself something that expresses this in a safer environment or with others who will keep you in check if you get too ahead of yourself.

Taurus – Embodying Venus' Feminine Nature

Taurus is an inert, earth-dominant, feminine sign. It is the natural second house of the zodiac, relating to possessions and food – the things in life that bring us a sense of comfort and security. This would also include a family who provide nourishment and clothing as well as a sense of belonging to a community. Both water and earth elements combine here to create a water-type individual. There can be a tendency to luxuriate too much in the body, creating an imbalance in weight or simply over-stimulation of the senses. Though this is, of course, your nature and should not be denied, it is also important here to be aware of the golden rule: When you are out of balance, you will seek things which further take you out of balance.

Balancing Taurus

If you are a water type, then it would be advisable to balance the need to luxuriate too much in any activity and get moving to break up any accumulated congestion or lethargy. With Venus' secondary 'airy' nature, there can be the tendency to want to skip over things in an avoidance of unpleasant emotions. It is important to feel everything that is coming up to be felt. This is the difference between avoidance and detachment. Avoidance means you cannot deal with a certain feeling whereas detachment shows an ability to feel it and yet not get carried away in the stories that develop from these feelings. This pleasure-seeking sign seeks pleasure with a steadiness (earth-dominant) and an ease (Venus) generally. This would have to be qualified by seeing if there are any planets in or influencing your rising sign. For example, if Saturn were placed in Taurus, then it would show more of an influence of air and any exercise would have to be modified to deal with the resulting dryness and possible anxiety. Once the planet that is placed in your rising sign has some form of expression, then the energy of the sign can be expressed with more ease.

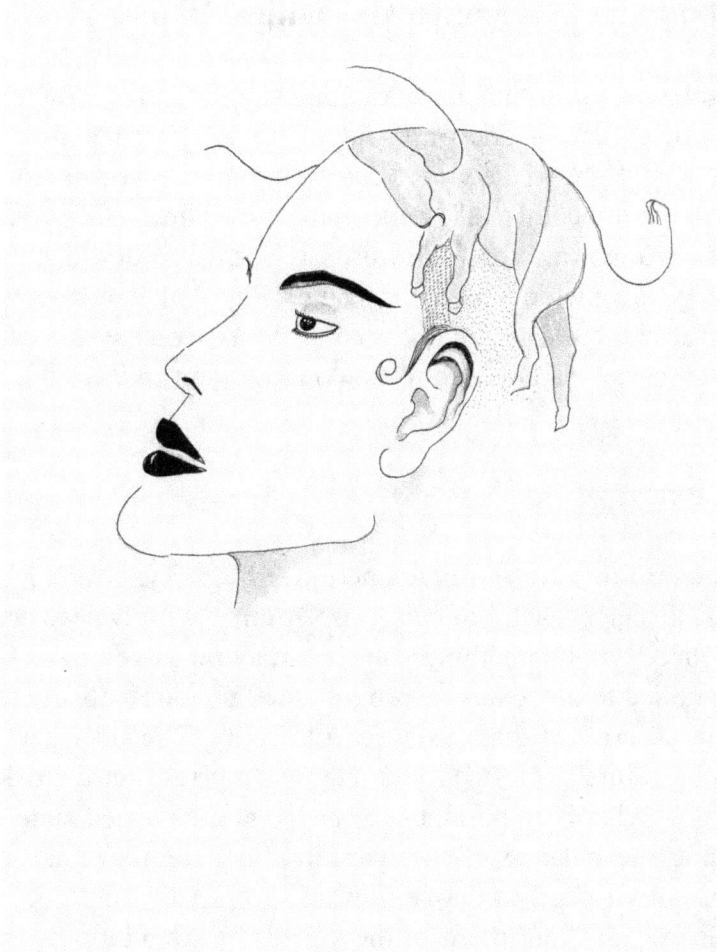

Taurus Body Parts

Taurus rules the face, mouth and throat. Tasting all of life's pleasures is not necessarily bad in and of itself. However, a life lived only on this level will not give you the fulfilment a higher connection can give you. Though you can be very content with your lot if there are no obstructing influences to your sign, there are joys beyond the body that are found by exploring this through the body itself. Exercise can be a first step in this exploration.

Gemini – Embodying Mercury's Masculine Nature

Gemini is a harmonious, air-dominant, masculine sign. It is the natural third house of the zodiac dealing with communication and interaction. It is ruled by the excitable and active planet Mercury. Here we see there can be a tendency for nervous disorders or, at the very least, a busy mind that leads eventually to dullness. This is due to its ruling planet Mercury. It is important for you to use the body in order to get out of your head. As you exercise, you quieten down the mind. Physical exercise will alleviate any nervous energy that can build up and will calm the nervous system. Getting more into your body in order to feel, as opposed to thinking all the time, would be the best advice for your sign.

Balancing Gemini

It might be beneficial for you to use the energy of Mercury, which represents the earth element, to practically approach your exercise routine with a need to learn something from it. Your intellect is not something you should avoid as you have a reasoning nature that needs to be applied to any exercise programme. You are unlikely to maintain such a programme if you do not see the reason for it! Taking a teacher's word for it will not satisfy your curious nature, so instead you may wish to test out the theories for yourself – in your own body. What is important is to arrive at a balanced state. Gemini is a dual sign and so finding the balance of the masculine and feminine is beneficial for you. When we exercise, we start to move inward eventually and, because the Gemini tendency is to always look out there in the world for stimulation, it would be a more profound connection when you look in and find that all you need in the way of stimulation is waiting for you there.

The other tendency for Mercury types is to be very impressionable, owing to the planet Mercury taking on the energy of the planets with which it associates. So choose your company carefully. Try to limit the amount of company you keep and how much information you expose yourself to. If you have chosen any type of activity from sports to training, you will be familiar by now with the fact that you must surround yourself with those who will encourage your routine. Fun can be experienced in a non-verbal interconnection with your fellow students in a class environment or with your fellow teammates. This frees up more energy from needless chit-chat – energy that is needed for your exercise.

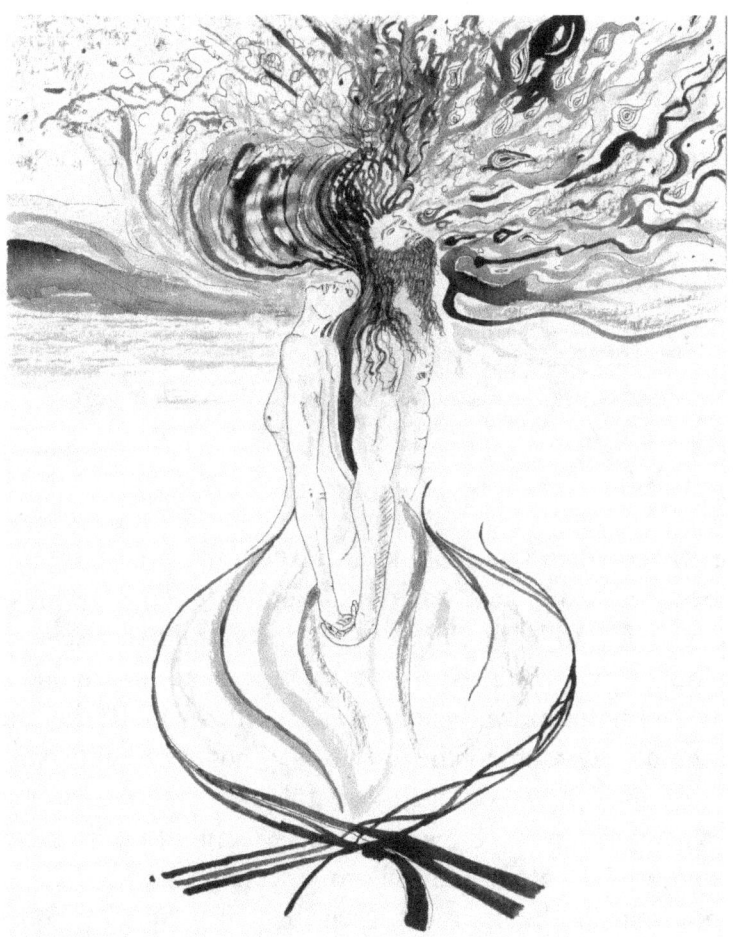

Gemini Body Parts

Gemini rules the neck, arms and hands. Your tendency is to look to all directions for further options, which only end up confusing you. Use the more concentrated focus of a certain point when exercising in order to stay focused on the task at hand. Above all else, have fun with any exercise you perform to express your curious, child-like energy.

Cancer – Embodying the Moon

Cancer is an active, water-dominant, feminine sign. It is the natural fourth house of the zodiac, dealing with the home and the mother – issues relating to comfort and well-being. It has water and air humours as it is a water-dominant sign and is ruled by the Moon, which is water-dominant when full and air-dominant when it is new. Therefore, it shows a mix of water and air depending on other indications. The Moon is the fastest-moving heavenly body, representing our ever-changing mind and emotions. Tuning into the cycles of the Moon is beneficial for you, as it is for us all. However, you may be swayed by moment-to-moment considerations more than other signs.

Balancing Cancer

Exercise can be initiated when you feel like it. Having the best of intentions in the world may not mean being able to stick to a set routine. This is because of the Moon's influence and the tendency to let feelings override physical exercise considerations. How you feel in the moment will sway your choices. So make the choice to exercise when and where you are feeling like it. Physical exercise allows all of the emotions to surface in a safe and peaceful environment in the body – not repressing anything or holding anything back. Everything must be felt fully in the moment. You do not have to express this verbally, as when you do there is a label on a feeling that is already passing. Your sign has a tendency to hold onto things and your feelings are no different. In actuality, a feeling that is not felt in the moment then becomes an emotion, which must be experienced at some time. Let them all go when you exercise your body. The mind and emotions are always in flux so it is important to develop a daily routine that can help still the mind in order to achieve a sense of peace in life. Once the stormy waters of the mind are calmed, it can reflect the true perfection in everything without the mind getting in the way. Use the body to still the mind.

The Moon represents the heart and can be accessed in gentle stretches that allow the heart to open slowly and safely. These are key considerations for your sign, which is always looking for safety and comfort. A gentle approach to your exercise and to yourself can facilitate this need. Exercise such as swimming can facilitate a gentle, yet more strenuous workout, in order to keep you in balance. When water is dominant, it would be beneficial to follow the water-balancing approach, especially if the Moon in your horoscope is waxing or full, i.e., moving away from or placed in opposition to your

Sun's position. However, if you also have Saturn in the first house, approaching exercise for an air constitution would benefit you as well. Your nature is still influenced by water, no doubt, but you will have to amend the routine to work with air. Remember that your constitution is a more complex thing than simply your rising sign. Here, the awareness would be on your sign's tendencies as well as your own unique expression of these. Saturn or the north node in Cancer will create all kinds of fears around the emotional body, so a gentle approach that allows for this will be more useful.

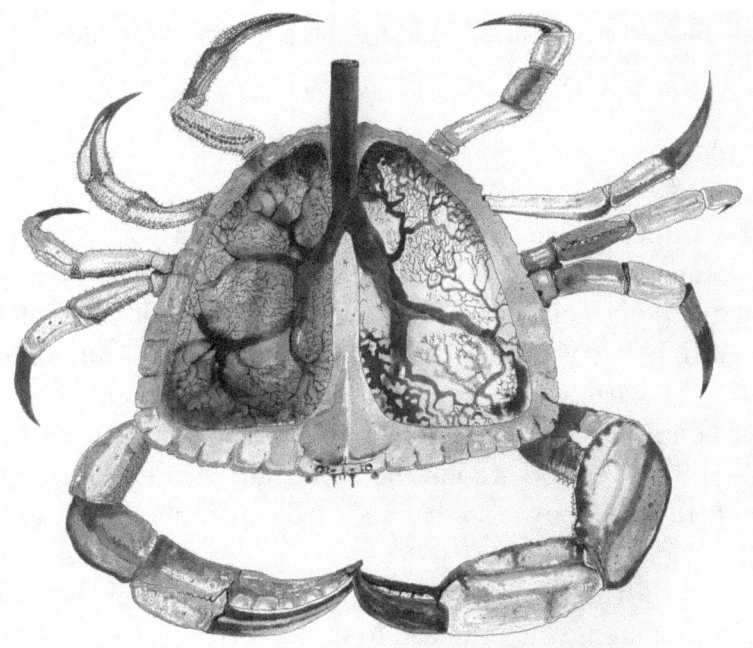

Cancer Body Parts

Cancer represents the heart, breast and lungs. Usually, your body type is more 'top heavy'. Exercises that do not address this will not bring balance. Cycling, for example, would not necessarily bring you complete balance, no matter how much of a workout you perform. A full range of body motion is needed, concentrating on the upper body, chest region and the arms. The arms are an extension of the heart and your ability to reach out to others. Though this is something you have a natural ability to do, you must also protect yourself. Finding strength in the arms through a workout will bring more of a solid foundation for your heart, allowing you to reach out in safety.

Leo – Embodying the Sun

Leo is an inert, fire-dominant, masculine sign. It is the natural fifth house of the zodiac, which represents creativity, children and games. The fullness we feel upon eating is expressed through this sign as a sense of being strongly self-centred. If Leo is your rising sign, then you are an embodiment of the Sun and can shine your warmth and generosity on others. You can also burn those around you with your self-centred approach. Your sign is fire-dominant and masculine in nature. Steadfastness and determination are your strengths.

Balancing Leo

Your nature is fire-dominant because of the Sun ruling, but you are less prone to injury than Aries, for example, because of a steadier approach. However, you would still ideally follow the fire-balancing approach and would benefit from allowing things to happen more than thinking you are all powerful and in complete control. We can fall into the trap of the ego when we believe we have achieved a goal, when in actual fact we have only allowed ourselves to come into alignment with our soul's purpose. You are an embodiment of the Sun, yet you are not the Sun itself! We are all tiny sparks from our great luminary. There is still power in that knowledge, but humility is also added into the mix.

The planets in Leo, if there are any, will also have a say in your nature. However, whatever exists in your sign, you will need to find a way to shine your bright light. Even an individual with Saturn in Leo will find it hard to deny their brightness once they have expressed the humility that is required. The Sun's energy needs to be expressed for you to feel healthy in physical form. Rhythm can be injected into your workouts, or any activity you perform, expressing the Sun's rhythmic nature. Leos may need to be more theatrical and in command in whatever they do and this can be facilitated by being the captain of a team, for example. If you have this tendency, then make sure your need for expression is not affecting others negatively in a class or team environment. Gradually, the intense glare of the Sun can be mellowed into a warm and passionate glow where you are encouraging to those around you.

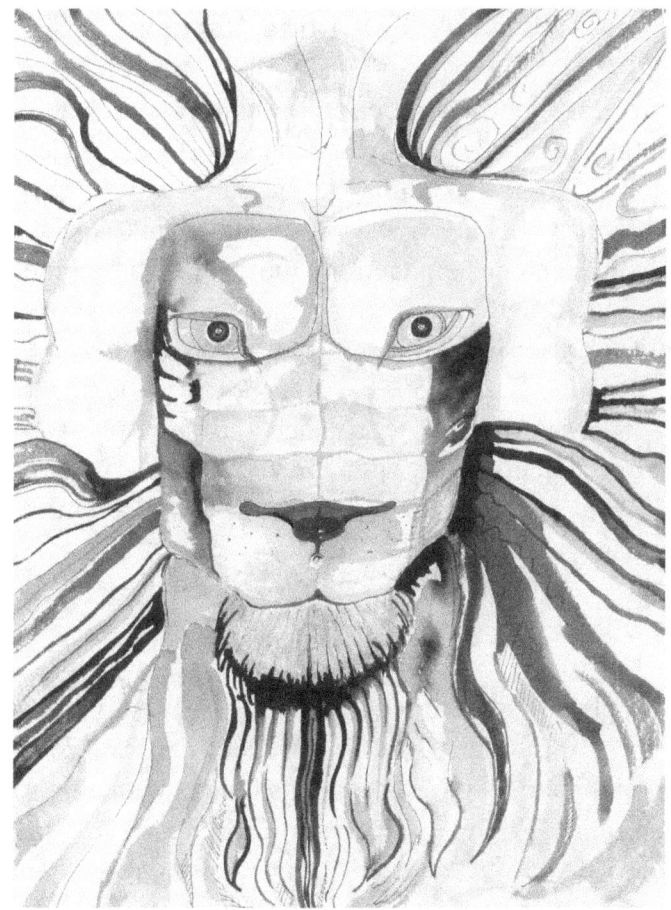

Leo Body Parts

Leo represents the heart (along with Cancer), as well as the region of the solar plexus, including the stomach, liver, gall bladder and spleen. Any exercises that address the mid-section would be beneficial, bringing in an adaptable range of motion. Following a fire-balancing approach to exercise may be appropriate unless there are other indications of air or water in your sign.

Virgo – Embodying Mercury's Feminine Nature

Virgo is a harmonious, earth-dominant, feminine sign. It is the natural sixth house of the zodiac, dealing with the elimination of disease, our debts and service to others. It is ruled by the impressionable Mercury so some of the same advice that applies to Gemini applies here also. Mercury finds expression in the outer world and its interactions through the masculine-oriented sign Gemini, but with Virgo, the journey is a more internal one as a feminine-oriented sign. Here, the task is to sort out that which does not work and eliminate it for your betterment. Virgo has the ability to take things apart and be very precise in how things are done in order to arrive at the best possible way of doing it. However, in order for you to balance the need to over-analyse, the advice would be to *feel* more if something is right for you or not. The strength of the intuitive impulse of Jupiter in your horoscope will indicate if this is a natural expression for you beyond simply your rising sign.

Balancing Virgo

You may wish to apply all of the theory that is necessary in order to achieve an understanding and then simply let it be. The tendency for Virgo is to want perfection because of a need to eliminate all of the problems but, as with any impulses of any of the signs, this can be overdone. Allow an expression of chaos sometimes in your activities and feel the energy move without the need for analysis always. Dance is a great way of achieving this balance. Having an earth-dominant sign as your rising sign as well as Mercury as your ruling planet shows an air and water nature if there are no other indications. Look to see if there are any planets in Virgo or in the other dual signs Sagittarius, Pisces and Gemini, to see which other expressions need an outlet through this sign.

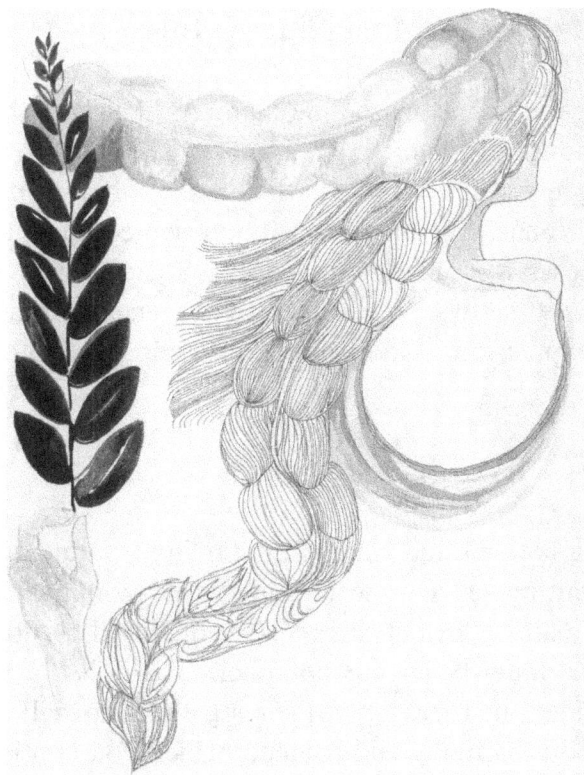

Virgo Body Parts

Virgo represents the lower abdominal region. Once the food has been ingested and felt as an enjoyment in the sign Leo, the sign Virgo is then about processing all that we have to digest. Exercises and routines that allow this process to work effectively and efficiently will express your Virgo nature. Yoga, martial arts and dance are great ways of achieving the precision in movement that your sign enjoys.

Libra – Embodying Venus' Masculine Nature

Libra is an active, air-dominant, masculine sign. As the natural seventh house of the zodiac, it represents how we relate to one another. The seventh house is our doorway into the world through our interaction with others. Libra is ruled by the planet of harmony and beauty Venus, but in a masculine-oriented sign, unlike Taurus, Venus' other sign. Taurus shows a more down-to-earth, practical expression of the pleasure principle whereas Libra shows Venus expressing itself in a more idealistic and expressive way. The expression of love and harmony is more intellectual in the air sign Libra.

Balancing Libra

Libra is seen as having both air and water humours in its nature and Venus is seen as an air- and water-dominant planet. Due to it being an air-dominant sign, Libra is seen as more dominant in air than water, but this must be qualified by other indications in your horoscope. An air- or water-balancing approach would be beneficial, depending on which is stronger. Planets in Libra or influencing the sign will impact your nature as always. Libra is all about harmony and balance, which you continually strive to obtain, whether in relationships, your work or your body. Venus shows a need to express oneself through art, so an exercise such as dance that is, at the very least, practised in an aesthetically pleasing environment is required. Soft furnishings and lighting will help set the mood for a love affair with your body. This sense of comfort in your routine will make an air type feel more cared for and make a water type feel right at home.

Try not to luxuriate too much in your body in whatever exercise you choose. Allow for some hard work to move energy. Saturn, the planet that represents a hard work ethic, finds its place of exaltation in your sign, so the possibility of applying yourself is always there. After the hard work is done, you can allow the body to settle in a nice long relaxation so that it can continue the balancing process. There is no need to intellectualise the process as the body knows best how to allow this harmony to occur naturally.

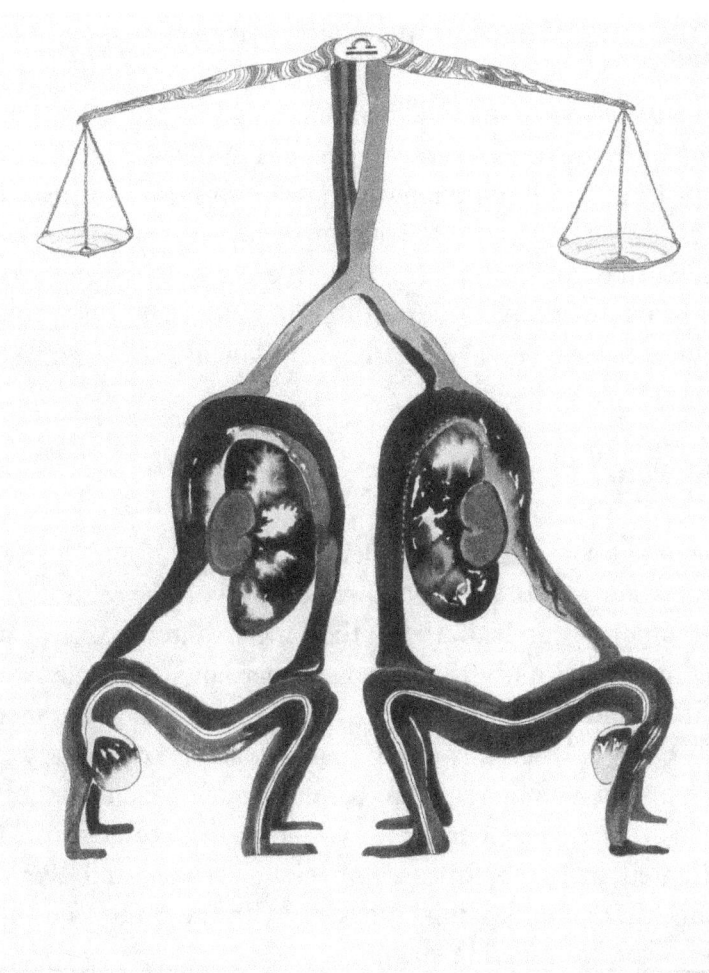

Libra Body Parts

Libra represents the pelvic region, the kidneys and the bladder. Venus represents the water element, which brings hormonal balance if it is well placed in the horoscope. The body achieves this without the need for our input all of the time. Even by breathing, our body is taking in what it needs and letting go of what is no longer needed, and in doing so, balancing the acidity and alkalinity in the body. Finding balance through dance, martial arts or yoga may be beneficial if this innate balance is lost for any reason.

Scorpio – Embodying Mars' Feminine Nature

Scorpio is an inert, water-dominant and feminine sign. It is the natural eighth house of the zodiac, dealing with transformation and sexual impulses. Mars finds its strength here in the depths of one's being, plummeting down through some stormy emotional waters at times. It is through the process of challenging negative emotions that you build up its strength and stamina in Scorpio. Its more negative traits are of manipulation and power games. These are Mars techniques in order to eliminate that which makes us feel weak. The intensity at which you delve deep may not always be expressed by your outer demeanour.

Balancing Scorpio

Being a water-dominant sign and being ruled by the 'fiery' Mars and Ketu makes you a mixture of fire and water – two elements that do not work so well together. This creates some antagonism, which needs an outlet in the form of intense exercise. Whenever there is a dual constitution, then follow the approach that suits the time of day, year and the stage of life. In the winter months through spring, there is a dominance of the water humour, so exercises to balance this energy are advisable, especially if you are a water type. During spring and summer, a fire-balancing approach can be developed. The nature of Scorpio is that of its ruler Mars, which is to take action. This Mars impulse needs to be facilitated in some form of physical activity and then transformed into something more opening and allowing. Working with the body frees up so much energy that may otherwise leave you feeling stagnant.

Scorpio energy can be quite intense as it is not only ruled by Mars, but it is also fixed in its purpose. There is a determination to see things through. This tendency must be allowed expression in order for it to soften in any activity. Otherwise, aggressive tendencies can prevail and injuries may result. The south node of the Moon is a co-ruler of your sign, showing the hidden aspects of your nature. Secret knowledge has a large part to play in the process of transformation. You may find yourself learning about unusual practices in order to remain in balance. Moving into a more intuitive space with your body will allow things to unfold gradually. The water humour needs constant stimulation, but when the fire humour is also present, it is advisable to take things at a steadier pace. As Confucius is quoted as saying, 'It does not matter how slowly you go as long as you do not stop.'

Notice the depth of your being that is beyond any turbulent emotions. Though the process of dealing with more challenging emotional upheavals may make you stronger in one sense, in another way we can see the stillness of your being as the most transformational experience that gives you all the strength you need. The intensity of your sign pushes you to achieve a great amount, be it extreme sports or through an inner journey of discipline and hard work, such as martial arts.

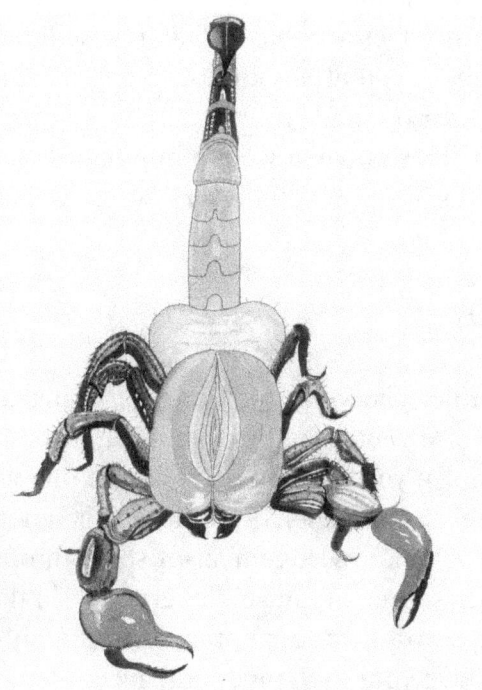

Scorpio Body Parts

Scorpio represents the genitals and the anus. These are the things in life we keep hidden and are not comfortable speaking about ordinarily. However, the need for this sign is to delve into the sex energy and cultivate it in order to transcend it. There is no denying the force of the sexual force, which is the life force. Any suppression is simply a fight with yourself and can only lead to a distortion of your energy. Scorpio needs to find an outlet for the strong sexual urge and one that will allow you to cultivate a more-balanced approach to all your activities. Otherwise the energy can move down and out, leading to a loss of vital energies that could otherwise add to a vibrant life.

Sagittarius – Embodying Jupiter's Masculine Nature

Sagittarius is a harmonious, fire-dominant, masculine sign. Jupiter's masculine expression creates high ideals. It is the natural ninth house of the zodiac, which represents the beliefs and guiding principles we live by. As a fire-dominant sign and its ruling planet being predominant in the water humour, it becomes more of a fire/water type if this is taken as the only factor at birth. This is a healthy type to be, but you must look at which energy is imbalanced at any time and approach activities according to the time of day, the current season and your age. The water humour is dominant in childhood and adolescence. This is when we are building the container of the body. The fire humour is dominant during our adult years when we are more goal-oriented in general.

Balancing Sagittarius

Jupiter being your sign's ruler shows a traditional, aspiring and idealistic approach to life. Approaching any exercise routine with more of an aspiration to reach higher states of awareness, beyond any form you identify with, can be one way this will express itself. Even a hatha yoga practice in and of itself would not be enough for such an idealistic individual. There must be an acknowledgement of spirit through a theoretical approach and a connection to a higher source organising everything in the universe. This may find expression through some type of devotional practice or simply devoting your practice to a guide or teacher who reflects your own inner guidance.

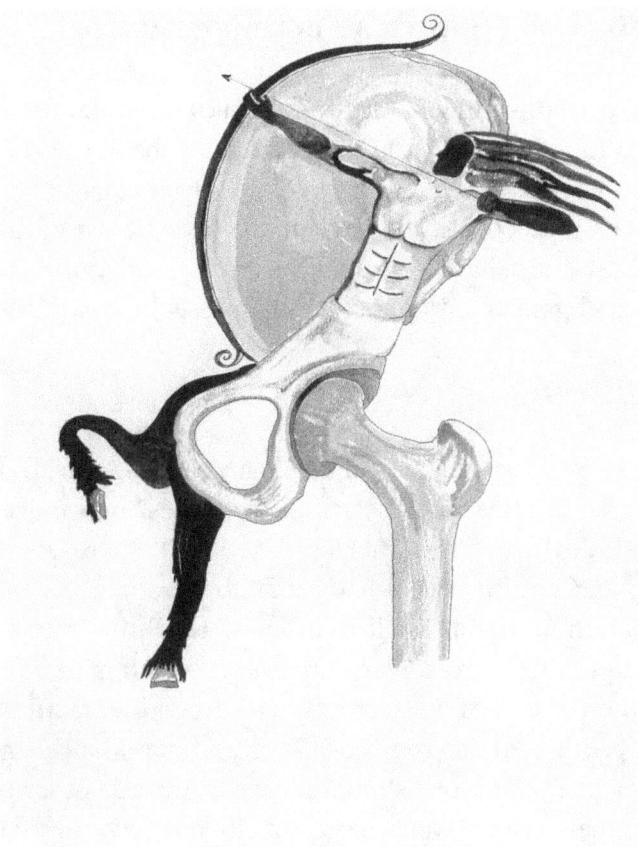

Sagittarius Body Parts

Sagittarius represents the hips and thighs. These parts of the body represent our firm foundations as we stand, giving us a clue as to the nature and strength of your sign. Having a strong belief in something is the best expression of this, and particularly if that something is beneficial to all concerned. Standing firmly in self-belief can help you balance stability with lightness and flexibility in the hips.

Capricorn – Embodying Saturn's Feminine Nature

Capricorn is an active, earth-dominant, feminine sign. It is the natural 10th house of the zodiac, which relates to the work we do in order to pay back our debts. It is ruled by the worker of the solar system, Saturn. Being an earth-dominant sign, we can see a water-type along with an air-type constitution when we take Saturn's influence into account. When air predominates, the wind blows and the earth is dried out. This will be modified by other indications and greatly influenced by the presence of a planet in your sign.

Balancing Capricorn

Capricorn is the hard worker of the zodiac. Whereas Sagittarius has an aspiration to achieve more idealistically, this impulse is put to the test in a more practical manner in Capricorn. Once the idealism of Sagittarius is reached, there comes a time when one must knuckle down and get on with what needs to be done. An image that is used for your sign is of a goat climbing up a hill in order to reach the top, although *Makara*, the Sanskrit name for Capricorn, means a 'sea creature', which is more likened to having the body of a goat and the tail end of a sea creature or crocodile. Hard work can certainly be facilitated in any physical exercise regime and Mars finds its place of exaltation here for this reason. However, the hard work should have no rewards other than being witness to the work itself. In other words, work hard but do not have any attachment to an end result. If an end result is all you are working for, then attachment results and pain will soon be snapping at your heels. In an air type, there is a detached approach and so the possibility of letting go in your work is there. You can also work on behalf of those who cannot do it for themselves. This may be facilitated through helping others achieve their best and the rewards of seeing your influence and hard work will be the payoff. Any exercise routine for Capricorn would ideally work with more standing exercises to gain a sense of stability in the legs and take some of the pressure off the back and shoulders.

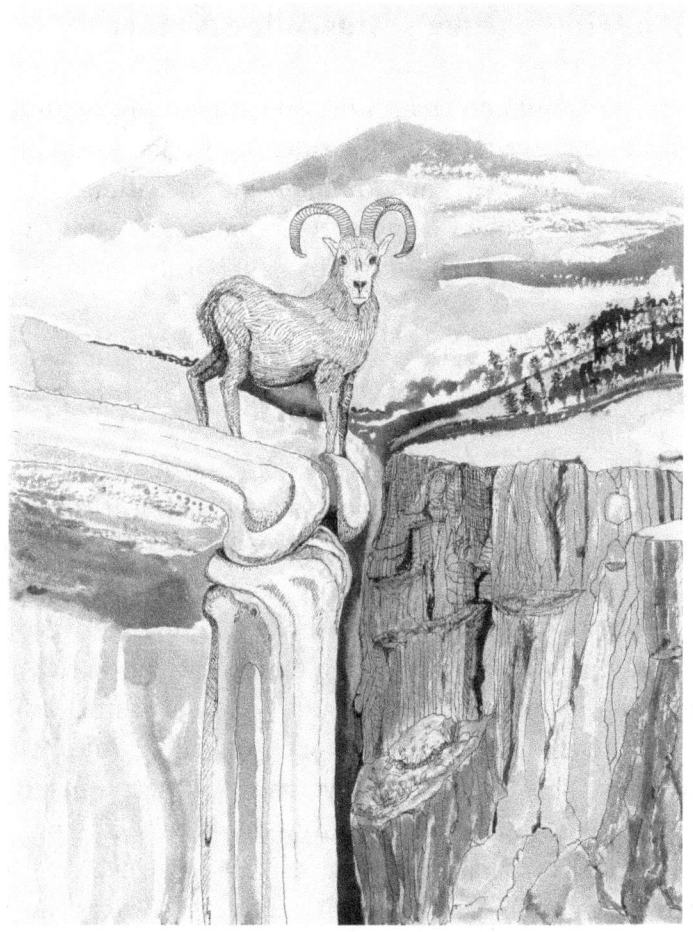

Capricorn Body Parts

Capricorn represents the back and the knees – two areas of the body that are required to work hard. If an individual is currently experiencing a Saturn period it can be felt in back and knee pain, as if holding the weight of the world on one's shoulders. The need to work hard and achieve a great deal can be facilitated by a more rigorous approach to physical work and exercise, but the ultimate goal is to detach from an end result. Saturn shows a capacity to work hard and let go of any attachments to the routine, or any of its benefits. Once you learn this lesson, all of the rewards from your hard work can come to you with more ease.

Aquarius – Embodying Saturn's Masculine Nature

Aquarius is an inert, air-dominant, masculine sign. It is the natural 11th house of the zodiac, which relates to our aspirations. It is ruled by both Saturn and the north node. It is an air-dominant sign, having two air-dominant planets ruling. It is also a more inert sign, with both of its ruling planets being inert in nature, as well as being a fixed sign. How does air become fixed? This is done by stubbornly upholding one's views and opinions.

Balancing Aquarius

The inert impulse of your sign needs to be acknowledged and worked with in any physical activity. This may be through working with slower exercises that allow the body to open slowly and ground the mind in your body. It may simply mean working with the physical body to create all of the insight and innovation you need in your life. Here the impulse is to take on a forceful role in developing and involving yourself with groups at large, but this may mean not paying enough attention to your own needs. The body can then suffer if it is not exercised enough. As your sign is air-dominant, it would be beneficial to stay with the body and the work will take care of itself sometimes. It is important for your sign to spend the time on yourself and see yourself as just as worthy a cause as you might be fighting for. The ability here is to see things very differently to everyone else and this can lend itself to great insights. However, with the air element, it is important to keep the mind under control or nervous disorders can dominate if you do not do any physical activity to balance it. Follow an air-balancing approach to exercise as outlined if this is your nature and allow the creativity to flourish in a safe environment.

Exercise for Aquarius could lead with more standing work as the lower legs are governed by this sign. However, unlike the conventional Capricorn, this sign's unusual needs can be facilitated through a more eclectic mix of exercises. Something unusual and thought provoking will stimulate your sign into more action and move from more inert pursuits that can lead to laziness and lethargy to more active pursuits. The goal of the practice should be ideally to bring you to a safe and secure resting period in your life, turning the mind off for a while and caring for yourself as you rest and recuperate.

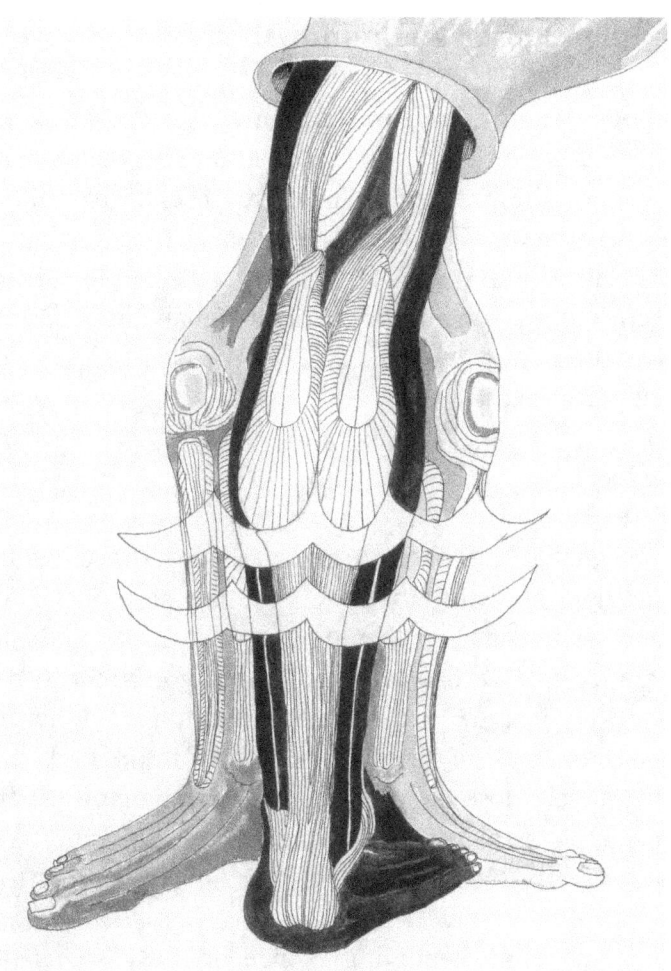

Aquarius Body Parts

Aquarius represents the calves, the shins and ankles. In your routines, you may wish to visualise your legs as solid trunks reaching down into the earth, grounding you in physical form. A tree can only grow as tall as its roots are deep. Keep this in mind when you are out there on the leading edge, paving new ground.

Pisces – Embodying Jupiter's Feminine Nature

Pisces is a harmonious, water-dominant, feminine sign. It is the natural 12th and last house of the zodiac, relating to letting go and liberation. Your sign is a water-dominant sign and its ruling planet, the prayerful Jupiter, represents the water humour. Here the water can be likened to an expansive ocean, where the undercurrents shift things around constantly. While in Cancer, the water is movable like a moving river that meanders and in Scorpio; it is fixed like a stagnant pool. This expansiveness can take everyone else's feelings and considerations above your own, so there is a need to address your own health issues with balanced exercises.

Balancing Pisces

Following a water-balancing approach to exercise as outlined would be beneficial for you if no other indications show otherwise. As the last sign of the zodiac, Pisces shows an individual looking beyond the reaches of everyday life. This can be expressed in a daily meditation practice and with a sense of letting go, being in the moment and one with it all. The practice of hatha yoga can help facilitate this letting go process. If a person is a water type, the tendency is to be more inert in the body and this can lead to a dulling of the mind. In order to overcome this tendency, one must first move through a more turbulent phase in physical exercise so as to move into a more relaxed, light feeling in the body. This allows you to sit comfortably for longer in order to ponder life's many mysteries.

Getting the body and energy moving is needed only so as to be able to sit in meditation and states of bliss for longer and longer. No dilly-dallying in yogic postures for hours on end for your sign. Get the body moving and the energy feeling lighter so that you can get to the real reason for your practice, which is your ability to sit in quiet awe and reverence. This will allow you to find balance and to express your harmonious nature.

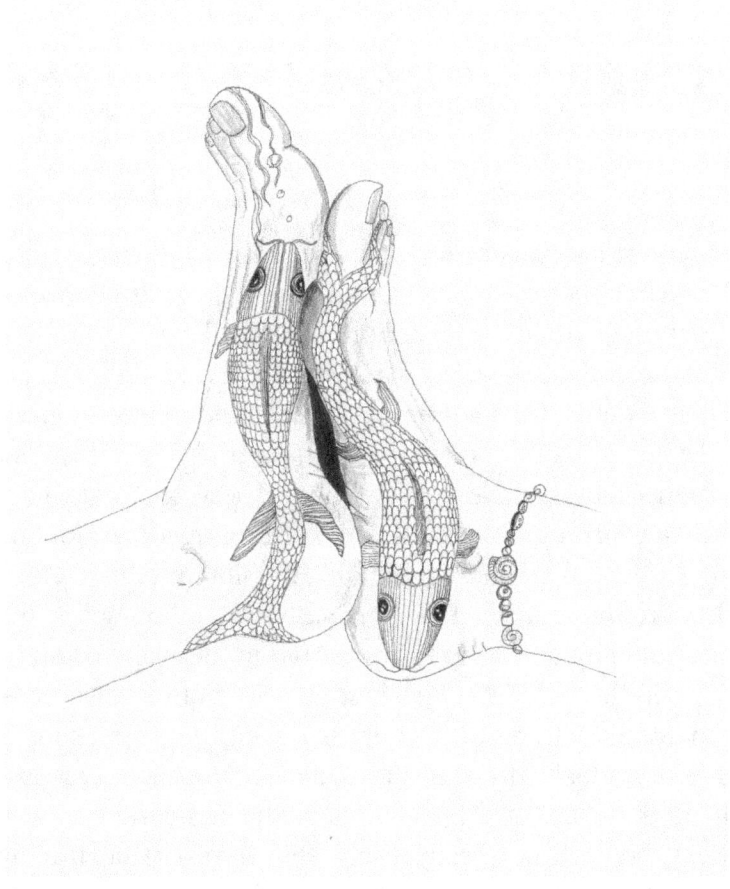

Pisces Body Parts

Pisces represents the feet. We often do not pay too much attention to the feet (unless maybe your sign is Pisces!) as we can disassociate with them often covered and furthest away from our heads. However, paying attention to the feet in any physical exercise brings us to a depth of being rarely experienced in our everyday lives. Any physical activity done standing can bring us into this awareness and away from any sense of disconnection in our own minds. It would be even better if you could do this barefoot in nature.

CHAPTER 7 – CHANGING PATTERNS

There are three layers of analysis in order to ascertain whether an imbalance will ripen for an individual, and whether this results in an illness or health concern of any kind that may adversely affect one's ability to exercise. The first layer is, simply, the promise has to be present in the horoscope. A seed has been sown and this will be reflected in the configuration of planets at birth. The second layer is the planetary period, which has to be in effect in order for it to produce its results. Whether these results are beneficial or not depends on many factors in the horoscope. These many factors are covered in *Essentials of Medical Astrology* by Dr. K.S. Charak, a medical doctor and the head of the Department of Surgery at the Indira Gandhi Hospital in New Delhi, India, as well as a renowned Vedic astrologer. According to Dr. Charak, 'a horoscope which is inherently strong does not indicate any suffering to the native in the wake of an ordinarily adverse *dasha*' (planetary period). Therefore, the first step in gaining awareness of any health-related issues is to see the strength of your rising sign and its ruling planet. The final layer of the cake is the transit of the planet which is in effect. This is the trigger in the horoscope. If all of these are not present, then the indication of a transit may only produce some effect, but will not bring results that have not been indicated from birth. On the other hand, if something is promised in the chart from birth, it is likely to manifest during the time period of a certain planet at some point in your life. This is, of course, within reason. If you are five feet tall as a fully grown adult, you are not going to be six feet tall at any point in your life, no matter how tall a time period or transit may say you are!

This book sets out to give some indication of constitution, which is only one layer of analysis, but a very important one in understanding your inherent strengths and ability to prevent or overcome any illnesses. The second layer is that of any imbalances as seen in planetary periods, which I will touch upon subsequently. The third layer of the transits is one which does not come under the scope of this book. However, this is one that is more likely to produce results if the first two layers are in place. In fact, if the promise is in your horoscope, you can be sure that it will produce some results at some point in your life. The planet promising to bring results will likely, at some point, begin its time period, and its transit will trigger these results at some point during that period. It is then simply a question of timing.

A Map for Living

Using the chart as a map, you can navigate through your life with more awareness. That is not to say that the entire route is clearly mapped out for us. We must use the knowledge gained by our observation of the stars with skill and have a sense of a bigger picture at play that we cannot always know. This is a balance that many who use astrology often fail to maintain as it is all too easy to wish to know as much as possible of what is to transpire. We must also give up the need to always know everything. That does not mean we do not prepare ourselves for a possibility. However, just because we have a reliable map does not mean we know what the destination will look like before we get there. We can only make estimations at best. We can know our overall path and make wise decisions on how to get there as smoothly as possibly, but we must also surrender to where life is ultimately taking us. Adding the awareness gained through the science of Vedic astrology can only increase the depth and experience in our chosen routines.

Planetary Influence

Planetary influences are activated during a planet's time period. These periods show what has now ripened for us to experience and promise the results of the thoughts, words and actions we have previously entertained. The results may be fixed, changeable or mixed in nature. The nature of these results for each individual is the work for an astrologer and is beyond the scope of this book. However, it is helpful to be aware of certain time periods. There are experiences that are fixed and will not change, except from our perspective once we have more awareness. There are others that are changeable and still others that are mixed in nature, offering mixed results. All of these benefit from our awareness and ability to accept each of them. One may look to see where the planet is bringing its imbalance, i.e., house position in the horoscope, and then see if the sign is inert, active or harmonious. In other words, is the result being experienced more fixed in nature, can we change it, or are there mixed results to be experienced?

Once a planetary period has been triggered in your life, the nature and qualities of that planet are pronounced in that time period. For example, if you are currently experiencing the period of Jupiter, then a more harmonious nature is pronounced if Jupiter is strong in your horoscope. You will be more interested in developing a broader knowledge base and begin to develop a connection to an inner guidance, possibly meeting teachers (including children), counsellors or advisers of some kind in order to facilitate this. The position and strength of the planet Jupiter at the time of your birth will show whether this will be an easy endeavour, and if the indications of Jupiter will be effortless or not. A weakness of Jupiter will show a difficulty in expressing these qualities, but an interest in them nonetheless. If you enter a Mars time period, you will no doubt develop a competitive streak, but whether you win or not is based on the strength and position of Mars in your horoscope. Each of the planets represents specific areas of our life, depending on what areas (houses) they rule in each individual's horoscope, as well as having general significations.

The planetary period you are currently experiencing will also impact the area of life it was placed in when you were born. If you have the planet Jupiter placed in, or influencing, your first house then Jupiter will express itself through your body more at that time. Whether this is experienced as an imbalance or not will depend on the strength of Jupiter and influences upon it as well as your constitution from birth by looking at other influences on your rising sign. An individual who is more of a water type will experience more imbalances due to Jupiter's influence on the first house during its time period than an individual with an air-type constitution. Any planet that has an influence on your first house, or your first-house ruling planet, will impact your physical body in some way during its time period. You should be able to correlate your findings in this chapter with your findings in the Ayurvedic form you filled out in Chapter Two, when keeping your current life experience in mind.

Special Influences

Certain aspects that assert a special planetary influence become active during that particular planet's period. The three outer planets Mars, Jupiter and Saturn have their own special sight in the horoscope. These are as follows:

Jupiter influences the 5th and 9th houses from where it is placed.
Mars influences the 4th and 8th houses from where it is placed.
Saturn influences the 3rd and 10th houses from where it is placed.
Rahu influences the 5th, 9th and 12th from where it is placed (counting anticlockwise).

All of the planets, as well as the Sun and Moon, influence the sign directly opposite (7th house) to where they are placed in the chart. Always count inclusively from the planet in question to the house in question, e.g., Jupiter in Taurus will influence the 5th, 7th and 9th houses from Taurus, i.e., the signs Virgo, Scorpio and Capricorn. These special influences are active during the planets' periods. However, there is always a time when these planets are activated on some level or other, so it is beneficial to add this awareness to the picture you have built up thus far. Examining your horoscope again, you can add this piece in order to see if there are any planets opposite to your rising sign that will be activated in that planet's time period. Look to see if Mars, Jupiter or Saturn has an influence on your rising sign or your Moon sign, based on these special influences. This will give you more of an indication as to any current imbalances as a result of the planet's period. The influences on your rising sign will be of a physical nature whereas those on your Moon sign will be of an emotional nature. Of course, this will have an impact on your physical health also.

Ever-Changing Nature

No matter what time period we may enter in life, if we are strongly influenced by a particular nature from birth, these periods will only modify this indication. A person who is only interested in feeding, sleeping and gathering material possessions is more influenced by the more inert planets Saturn and Mars as well as the north node of the Moon. The planets Saturn, Mars and the north node represent laziness, selfish desires and greed. Though such an individual may move through all of the planetary influences in their life, and become influenced by the Sun, Moon and Jupiter and their more harmonious influences, they may not express this balanced nature as much as someone with more of a harmonious nature from birth. These harmonious planets may be placed in weakness and obstructed in some way. An example of this may be a criminal who plots and schemes in the background (north node) and then involves others in his scheming in order to gain as much money (Mercury) and the resulting pleasures (Venus) due to his takings. These are all selfish pursuits. Although this person may become more concerned for others' welfare at some point in life, e.g., when a Moon period is active, they may not express as much altruism as a person with an inherently altruistic nature would express during this time period.

Another example would be someone who is born with a more altruistic nature. This person may live an altruistic life in one sense or another throughout their life, but there will be times in their life when more selfish concerns are dominant. An example of this would be a Saturn period, where the individual may become ill and have no choice but to look after his or her own needs. Only a saintly individual would continue to consider others before themselves – even as they suffer an illness. These inherent natural forces are always influencing us at varying degrees. We access these all of the time, but our natural urges and tendencies will lean more towards one or the other depending on what our horoscope indicates.

Planetary Periods and Health

In Vedic astrology, planetary periods are studied in order to understand that which is unfolding at any given time for an individual. They represent a timeline of our lives which show the results of past thoughts, words and actions that are ready to be experienced at present, and whether these results will be experienced as positive or negative. Seeds have been sown in the past and whatever fruit has been planted, you would expect that fruit to be produced. In this way, we can see the ripening of these results in planetary periods. Today we have the use of computers to calculate these periods, but in ancient times these time cycles were intuited by the sages of India. These periods are perfect in their progression and show the natural time cycles and development of the spirit, mind and body throughout life. There are many planetary periods that are studied depending on the specifics of the horoscope. However, the main one that is used universally, and which can be applied to any horoscope, is the 120-year life span analysis.

Each planetary period increases a certain quality that is either inert, active or harmonious. Whether this increase brings health issues will depend on whether a certain quality being experienced at any given time is balancing to your overall quality. For example, if you were born with more inert qualities, leading to a dulling of the mind and body, then entering into a period that increases this dulling effect will increase this quality and will likely lead to ill health. Ill health may be experienced as simply a lack of vitality through a lack of movement or through a debilitating illness. However, if a more active individual enters a more inert period, or vice versa, then balance is possible for that individual.

In order to see periods that would indicate an actual illness, there are many factors that need to be taken into account. One such factor is a period of the planets which rule either your 2nd, 6th, 7th, 8th or 12th houses in your horoscope, particularly the 6th or 8th houses in relation to ill health. These may bring up health issues that may or may not lead to an illness. You may wish to look after your health and cultivate healthy lifestyles and habits during these periods. If your ruling planet, i.e., the planet that rules your first house, is strong in your horoscope, then you have the ability to withstand many imbalances and you may not experience an illness as a result, or you may experience mostly good health with an occasional illness. During a period of your first-house ruling planet, you may be more concerned about health issues in general, whether or not you experience this as illness.

Retrograde Planets and Health

A planet that appears as if it were moving backwards from our perspective on Earth is known as a retrograde planet. If the planet that rules your first house is retrograde, it can bring up health issues which need to be dealt with. This is particularly pronounced during the planet's time period. Having a retrograde planet as your ruling planet does not, in and of itself, mean you will have an illness. However, there may be some issues to deal with regards to your health during its time period. It may be that you always seek to find an elusive balance in your health routines and this may provide you with a struggle to find this balance in your life.

Imbalances

Pay attention to the element of the planet you are currently experiencing in a planetary period analysis. If you already have a predominance of a particular element in your own makeup, it would be beneficial to take this awareness with you through these time periods. This will allow you to more consciously balance the tendency to experience an excess, and subsequent imbalance, of this element during the planet in question's time period. If, for example, you are in a period of Mars and you are a fire type, then there is more of a likelihood that you will need to address an excess amount of fire during Mars' time period and any resulting imbalances. The house position of Mars will dictate where you experience these imbalances. If Mars also rules your 6th house, then an illness is more likely as this is an area of possible weakness along with the 8th house.

The 6th house, and its ruling planet, brings illness due to our own bad habits and lifestyle choices. Our awareness of its time period can be very helpful in dealing with any negative effects. The 8th house, and its ruling planet, shows illnesses that are chronic in nature and more difficult to treat. These conditions often worsen during a period of the 6th or 8th house ruling planet, or periods of planets located in your 6th or 8th house. Again, the strength of your first-house ruling planet will show whether or not you can cope with this illness. The timing of these illnesses is calculated using the planetary periods and a trigger transit of the planets in question.

For an understanding of any health-related results for you at present, you can keep an eye on the time period of any planets that are placed in your first house, and its time period, as well as the time period of any planets that influence your first house or a planet that rules your first house. The 6th house of health can also be looked at to see health-related issues as well as any planets that are either placed in your 6th house or influence your 6th house. Use all of the techniques for analysing your 6th house as you did for your first house in order to come to conclusions about this influential planet on your health and well-being. The 8th house and its ruling planet can then also be studied for health-related issues.

Three Layers of Analysis

The major periods span many years and show what we are currently developing in our lives as well as the general circumstances we find ourselves in. These time periods show what is being experienced, taking a look at the bigger picture and at our soul's journey. These cycles can also be studied in relation to phases within these longer time periods and show how we are feeling about these circumstances as well as the people we are meeting to teach us something along the way. These sub-periods, which are represented by the level of mind and emotions, are more relevant to our lives, as we experience life more directly by how we feel. Within these periods, we can study a shorter time period that shows how we are using our intelligence and how we are reacting to where we find ourselves within these longer time cycles. These three levels represent the spirit, mind and body.

To experience all of the major periods in our lives, we would have to live for 120 years. This is the sum total of all the major planetary periods added together before they would begin to repeat themselves. Using the sub-periods, we can see that these cycles repeat themselves throughout our lives. This is why we have patterns we live with throughout our lives, though these patterns alter, according to other longer time periods we experience at various stages of our life. In other words, different faces and different places may come and go in our lives, but we have familiar experiences throughout our lives.

The Nine Planetary Periods

This knowledge can be used in conjunction with a more static analysis as seen in your horoscope, showing a more dynamic experience throughout life. You were born with a certain eye colour, for example, so no matter what the time period suggests, you will remain blue eyed if that is the colour your eyes have always been. However, the quality of your eyesight may change. There are certain things that are constantly changing, such as your lifestyle and weight, and most certainly your mind and emotions. This type of dynamic analysis can be looked at using the planetary periods and their dominating quality, in order to come to a deeper awareness of your nature in the time period you are currently experiencing. You may also wish to pay attention to a planet's influence on your Moon sign, as its time period begins, to see the influences on your mental and emotional health. This will, of course, affect your physical health in some way. For example, if you are currently in a Saturn period of life, and Saturn has an influence on your Moon through the 3rd, 7th or 10th houses, then the increase of air is relevant and may result in anything from debilitating fear to joyful detachment, depending on the position of Saturn in your horoscope. In the case of someone who is dominant in the air humour from birth, and is currently experiencing a Saturn period, then it will more than likely find its expression through fear. However, finding a more balanced expression of air can be reached, which can lead to a joyous detachment in a Saturn period.

The Nine Major Time Periods

The South Node - 7 years
Venus - 20 years
Sun - 6 years
Moon - 10 years
Mars - 7 years
The North Node - 18 years
Jupiter - 16 years
Saturn - 19 years
Mercury - 17 years

Though there is a natural order to these cycles, we each begin at different stages and experience these at various periods in our lives. Each period has general significations, though we each experience these in our unique way. It is an astrologer's job to shed light on your unique path and experience of these periods. In order to observe your current place in these time cycles, and your own timeline, you must have a Vedic birth chart calculated for your exact time of birth. An approximate time of birth will give you an approximate timeline.

A South Node Time Period

The natural beginning of these time periods (though not necessarily yours) begins with the south node (Ketu) - the 'shadowy planet'. Ketu represents the tail end of the serpent in Vedic myth, the headless part of the mythic demon Vasuki, opening us up to past life connections and bringing us into the realm of spirit. It can be a confusing and challenging time, as it dissolves things on a material plane in order to bring us to that sense of spirit. The south node is a part of us that is aware that we are pure spirits in physical form and nothing in this physical existence can live up to that ideal. The south node is a calculated point on the ecliptic, as opposed to a physical planet. It operates on a psychological level and is, for the most part, difficult to comprehend. An eclipse can obscure and dull the mind and our true nature, but this can also illuminate us once the earthly dissatisfaction and confusion is experienced.

Generally, a south node period would increase the fire humour in one's life experience. The results of this would depend on its unique role for you in your horoscope. However, overall the quality of dullness can at times lead to breakthroughs, like breaks in the clouds. Follow a fire-balancing routine in order to dispel any build-up of toxic heat. Often, the nature of any illness experienced during the south node's time period is difficult to understand and treat. This is the obscuring nature of an eclipse.

A Venus Time Period

After a period of rejection, or challenges, with materiality during the south node period, we enter a phase that brings us back into contact with our sensual desires once again. We begin to seek out pleasures, especially if we are strongly influenced by the planet Venus from birth. The water element gives and sustains life. In its period, Venus gives us an appreciation of the finer things in life. As a tourist guide to our more material pursuits, Venus represents our physical desires that need to be acknowledged in its time period. Water smoothes all of life's rough edges, so Venus represents the need to sensitise to others' needs as well as our own. Venus is an active planet so our desire is to taste life during its period. Both air and water can increase and this can be seen in an increase of movement and interaction as well as indulgence, especially if it is strongly influencing your first house. This impulse would need to find balance with more activity or may lead to imbalances such as laziness and lethargy.

A Sun Time Period

After a period of pleasure within a Venus period, and perhaps a time when we overindulge, we enter into a period of the Sun to begin the purification process. Sun bathing naturally detoxifies us. However, too much Sun can also burn, so we can see how during a Sun period we may burn others who get too close – burning away any perceived imperfections. The Sun is, after all, a representation of spirit and is not so concerned with sensual pleasures. The impulse here is pure, where we wish to discover our true sense of power.

Depending on the strength of your Sun, this time can be one of gaining power and confidence in the world, as you tune into your true sense of Self, or it may be a period to feel the weakness of your lost connection to source, spending the time needing to work on your self-esteem and self-confidence. The greatest sense of confidence comes from a connection to your true spirit. You can then shine this light generously on others. The Sun will generally increase the fire humour and, if well placed in the chart, it will lead to a balance of fire. This is expressed as robust health and vitality. However, if the Sun is weakly placed, there can be a lack of fire and a subsequent loss of digestive ability and vitality as well as all the ramifications of a lack of these.

A Moon Time Period

After a period of connecting to one's Higher Self in a Sun cycle, we once again connect to others and their needs in a Moon period. The Moon represents the heart and our need to put down roots and connect and care for others. It is a time in our lives where we look to be nourished by others and wish to offer the same nourishment in return. Food, family, community and a sense of belonging are all expressions of a Moon period, though each individual will find their unique way of experiencing this comfort. It can be a changeable period, as seen in the changing phases of the Moon, reflecting the ever-changing nature of the mind and emotions. If your Moon is waxing or full, there is an increase in the water humour and the resulting effects of heaviness or congestion may be present if it strongly influences areas of health and the body. If your Moon is waning or new, the air humour increases and must be balanced in order to avoid a feeling of lack.

A Mars Time Period

Mars begins a period where we are more concerned with our own sense of power in the world. It represents our need to strengthen ourselves and express our individuality. After a Moon period, Mars draws us away from others and brings us a need to look after our own interests once again. Becoming a leader in your field or going it alone are very much Mars-type experiences. Finding your strength, whether physically or emotionally, is represented by Mars. Mars is the warrior, showing our ability to suffer discomfort in order to progress in a routine. In order to get up and exercise, Mars needs to be strong. Mars represents our needs which need to be fulfilled if we are to destroy our weaknesses. This is a time period that disconnects us from others, bringing us more of an experience of selfishness into our lives. This is often a destructive time period, representing a necessary destruction of those things in life that weaken us, be they bad habits, lifestyles or company.

Fire increases in Mars' time period, increasing competitiveness. If Mars strongly influences your first house or its ruling planet, then this fire will dominate and imbalances are possible unless the fire is counteracted by influences that cool down your system. Toxic heat conditions may be present with anger and/or a need to control events and people in your life. Even a strongly placed Mars can bring imbalances of toxic heat as Mars is a malefic planet.

A North Node Time Period

In a period of the north node, life gets interesting and can feel like we are living on the edge. In fact, that is exactly what occurs, as we are pushed out to the fringes of life in order to find a new and exciting way forward. Rahu, the north node of the Moon, represents the head of the serpent *Vasuki* in Vedic myth. The first bite from its mouth, and the beginning of a north node period, can bring with it the venom before settling down into what is, for the most part, a period of excess. Whereas the south node is the need to give things up on a material level, the north node is the need to experience life intensely, being the head of the serpent, and where we are to taste all that life has to offer. It can be a very exciting period in a person's life, but it can also be like a roller coaster ride that, after a while, becomes quite tiresome. There is a purpose for everything in life and the north node's purpose is to ultimately bring a sense of disillusionment with worldly experiences and achievements. It represents our soul's need to experience all that life has to offer that has not being satiated previously. Sometimes the mind and body are not willing or able to take the journey. It will ultimately give you the experience, but the lesson learnt is that nothing can ultimately satisfy us materially. This brings us back to spirit, but only after we have had our fill. The influence of the north node is of obscuring the light of the Sun and Moon. In other words, its time period represents a period of confusion as our ego pursues a path that obscures our connection to our true source of power.

The north node increases the air humour and brings out its more imbalanced expressions through irrational fears. Its effects are mostly psychological, unless it is influencing areas of health, but because of the impact on the mental and emotional body, it will often manifest physically as a psychosomatic condition. If the north node influences your first house, or first-house ruling planet, then it can increase a drying effect on your body. This will need to be acknowledged in order to counteract the possible imbalances of air, especially if you were born as an air type. The north node, just as the south node, shows illnesses which are difficult to diagnose, and therefore treat.

A Jupiter Time Period

After the intense life experience of the north node, we use the experience gained to develop a more even keel in a Jupiter period. Jupiter is the planet that gives us the ability to believe in something we cannot see, i.e., faith. We develop a faith in something that can bring us higher than the worldly experiences that the north node brought. Jupiter is a harmonious planet if well placed so it brings us a sense of connection to something greater than ourselves. If the north node made us disorganised, then Jupiter organises our lives once again and we are grateful for it. The north node period can be one where we paddle against the current, until Jupiter allows us to let go with the natural stream of life. Jupiter is the largest, most benevolent planet, bringing with it blessings and expansion in its time period. When we have a Jupiter experience, the result is always expansion in some way, but it is more profoundly a sense of our Higher Self and connection to a higher power within us that graces our lives.

The water humour can increase during a Jupiter time period if Jupiter strongly influences your first house or ruling planet. This can lead to an imbalance of the water element if Jupiter is strongly placed, which usually increases weight. This tendency can be counteracted with lifestyle routines that offer more adaptability and change to your exercise routine. A strongly placed Jupiter usually indicates good health overall, as it is the most benevolent planet.

A Saturn Time Period

After a period of expansion in a Jupiter period, we enter a period of Saturn where we have to slow down. We expanded as far as we are going to within a Jupiter period and during a Saturn period, we experience a reality check. This period shows a need to let go of something in order to move on, feeling lighter afterwards. The letting go part is sometimes the hardest lesson Saturn has to teach, but is one that offers the greatest rewards. However, that is not to say that Saturn is a time to sit back and relax. It is a time to work hard and commit to something that is worth working towards. Anything that is worthwhile will only come to us if we are willing to work hard with consistency. Once we learn this lesson, we can let go of always wanting to see instant results. Saturn does not give fast results. All that we have strived for will come in time and all that needed to be let go of will be taken away if we have not been able to release our grasp. This period is more inert in general and pulls us away from others in order to protect ourselves. Fear is usually how Saturn is experienced. The Sanskrit name for Saturn is *Shani* and comes from the same Sanskrit root word *Shanti*, meaning 'peace'. Here we can see that we need to make peace with the fact that one day we will lose everything and everyone, before finally losing our physical body to the death experience. We can only say we are truly at peace when we have accepted this.

Inevitably, we will experience an increase of the air humour in a Saturn time period. This is especially true of those born an air type and who have Saturn strongly influencing the first house, ruling planet or Moon. However, we all experience Saturn's drying effect somewhere in our lives, as Saturn is the primary planet of disease. Look to see where Saturn is placed in your own horoscope to see what area of the body is affected by illness. To counteract this tendency, one must develop strategies for the air element, acknowledging its presence in our life, but working with it in more productive ways. Saturn has an inert quality that we must keep moving in a steady, considered fashion in order to remain physically and emotionally well. You may need to purposefully invite pain into your life in order to express this quality. This may be achieved through a strict exercise programme and healthy lifestyle routines. It is far better to experience the pain of working out than the pain of illness due to a lack of exercise. Emotions need to move through us also or they become logged in the body as pain. Saturn's period brings these up as a physical and emotional detox.

A Mercury Time Period

After the slow lessons that are taught by Saturn, the slowest planet, we come into a period of Mercury, the fastest-moving planet. Mercury represents our intellect and shows the speed at which our thoughts travel. In a Mercury period, we become child-like once again, after having learnt the sometimes difficult lessons Saturn had to teach us. Mercury makes us curious about life and is a time when we seek others out to play with. The word 'curious' has its roots in a word meaning 'to heal'. After Saturn disconnected us from others and from a feeling of well-being, Mercury gets us to integrate the experience and heal. We are emptied of anything unnecessary in a Saturn period so that we can make room to be curious about life in a Mercury period. Mercury represents this need to learn something new. We develop skills with Mercury and become experts if Mercury is strong, allowing us to work in our chosen field. Learning something new re-wires our brains and allows something new to be born within us. In a Mercury period, we can develop a more light-hearted approach to life, as it is the most emotionally detached impulse. Mercury is also the closest planet to the Sun and our true power, so after a period of feeling the farthest away from our power in a Saturn period, we now come back and can integrate the experience in a Mercury period.

The humour that is increased in Mercury's time period very much depends on the position and influences upon Mercury in your horoscope. It does increase activity overall and may lead to all kinds of nervous disorders if not balanced with relaxation techniques. You may need to cultivate more relaxation if you are to counteract this planet's stimulating nature.

Patterns within Patterns

Once we have applied ourselves in the world again and gained a more practical approach to living in a Mercury period, it naturally follows that a south node period will bring us back into our true spirit, which is not concerned with worldly achievements. After a Mercury period, the south node begins the cycle again. On it goes, over and over, we experience these natural time cycles throughout our lives on many levels – from minute to minute, hour to hour, day to day, month to month and year to year. Each cycle that repeats does so in a new environment, as expressed in other concurring periods, and through the ever-changing transit of these planets. So it can be seen that we experience similar patterns but within different circumstances, and with different people and events guiding us. The circumstances are represented by the major planetary periods that do not repeat themselves (unless you live to the ripe old age of 120!). The sub-periods repeat themselves over the years for anything up to three years in length, although sometimes only for a few months at a time. Even though environments and faces in our lives change, the patterns of our life are always familiar.

Discovering Your Timeline

We each find a unique expression of these cycles in our lives according to our own unique horoscope. With the knowledge of Vedic astrology more accessible now more than ever before in history, we can become aware of a new phase beginning and can work with letting go of old ways of being. The benefit of knowing where we are in relation to these time cycles, and understanding our own timeline, is that we learn to release resistance to the natural flow and our life's natural unfolding. This allows us to experience a greater sense of ease in life and in our bodies.

We can then begin to grab opportunities in time periods that are more conducive to the quality being expressed. Whether we are in a period that is more inert, active or harmonious, we can begin to accept and work with any period in our lives to begin to find balance overall. By learning to accept these qualities throughout life, we can make the most of our experience as spirit that has taken form for a life experience.

Boats on an Ocean

The transit system is a dynamic analysis that looks at the current transit of the planets and how they are bringing you towards your destination. Together the transits and periods of planets show your ever-evolving life experience. This phenomenon can be explained using the analogy of our horoscope as a boat on an ocean – an analogy Pearl Finn used to teach. The boat has the wind blowing its sails and the undercurrents taking it along. The boat is our horoscope, or the results of previous lives lived that have brought us to where we are now. The winds are the transits of the planets that are either pushing against where we want to be or taking us even faster to where we are going. The sea is the time period we are experiencing that shows what is coming up from within for us to experience at any given time. Ultimately, the sea will have its way with us, but may or may not be assisted by current transits.

When you have an awareness of these influences, you have an awareness of where you are on the vast ocean that is your life. This awareness automatically brings a sense of ease with whatever is going on in your life. If you know a period of time for you is going to be physically or emotionally challenging, then you know to batten down the hatches and ride it out with the tools at your disposal. At the very least, knowing when a period is beginning and ending brings an enormous sense of peace, no matter what has to be faced. You can also take full advantage of the winds that are taking you out of the choppy waters and to calmer seas. This means knowing a time period that is beneficial for you is worked with more consciously and deliberately to gain maximum benefit from it. This may be scheduling some time off if necessary, or sticking to a more dynamic physical exercise programme. If you put the work into any activity, be it a physical exercise routine or any improvement on yourself, you will of course reap the benefits with consistency over time. However, you do yourself a great service by accepting your fate and moving toward creating more beneficial actions for your unique body type and nature. This awareness allows you to react according to the planets that have an influence on you. By using the best of what you have under your belt, and the best of what you are developing, you create an environment in which you can thrive.

Afterword

The gift of Vedic astrology is to know and accept our limitations, while at the same time taking full advantage of the cosmos in order to achieve something that is achievable at present. Knowing your physical limitations is as important as knowing where your strengths lie. You must limit yourself and focus your energy in order to work at something, including an exercise routine. The great benefit of having an awareness of the influence of the planets is the ability to move with helpful influences, timing appropriate routines. Of course, this is all to be taken in context. Just because a certain time period shows it is more conducive to work with something does not mean that whatever that may be is something you have within you to achieve. Just because a time period is showing that a more physical expression is needed does not mean you were born to be a pro-athlete. You will find your way to an exercise programme and capability within your scope. Everything must be taken into context when looking at planetary periods and transits as each and every one of us experiences them in our own unique way.

No one can actually give us a complete sense of that which is unfolding for us at any given time. Someone who is proficient in the language of the stars can, of course, give you a good idea, but that is all. You are the one living it and you must become your own guide if you are to develop this sense of acceptance of the possibilities within your limitations. Working within your destiny is a necessary restriction in the sense that this limitation focuses you and allows you to apply your free will in the context of being able to achieve all that is achievable at any given time.

My wish is that this book gives you a sense of how perfect you are, just the way you are, and in making any improvements, that everything is happening perfectly. Anything you do is simply adding to your perfection, playing your part in the greater whole which is perfect.

References

Bhagwan, Dr. R.K. and Dash. *Caraka Samhita Vol. 1.* (tr.) Sharma, . Varanasi, India: Chowkhamba Sanskrit Series Office, 2006, pp.34.

Charak, Dr. K.S. *Essentials of Medical Astrology.* New Delhi, India: UMA Publications, 1994, p. 95.

deFouw, Hart and Svoboda, Robert. *Light on Life: An Introduction to the Astrology of India.* New Delhi, India: Penguin Books India, 2006, p. 33.

Frawley, David and Summerfield Kozak, Sandra. *Yoga for Your Type.* 3rd ed. New Delhi, India: New Age Books, 2001, p. 8.

Larsen, Visti. *Jyotish Fundamentals.* New Delhi, India: Sagittarius Publications, 2005, p. 155.

Rath, Sanjay. *Vedic Remedies in Astrology.* New Delhi, India: Sagar Publications, 2000, p. 395.

Sharma, G. S. *Brihat Parasara Hora Shastra. Vol. 1.* (tr.) New Delhi, India: Sagar Publications, 1994, pp. 28-29.

Sutton, Komilla. *Personal Panchanga and the Five Sources of Light.* Bournemouth, England: The Wessex Astrologer Ltd., 2007, p. 25.